Lecture Notes in Computer Science 9534

Commenced Publication in 1973
Founding and Former Series Editors:
Gerhard Goos, Juris Hartmanis, and Jan van Leeuwen

More information about this series at http://www.springer.com/series/7412

Oscar Camara · Tommaso Mansi
Mihaela Pop · Kawal Rhode
Maxime Sermesant · Alistair Young (Eds.)

Statistical Atlases and Computational Models of the Heart

Imaging and Modelling Challenges

6th International Workshop, STACOM 2015
Held in Conjunction with MICCAI 2015
Munich, Germany, October 9, 2015
Revised Selected Papers

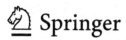 Springer

Editors

Oscar Camara
Universitat Pompeu Fabra
Barcelona
Spain

Tommaso Mansi
Siemens Corporation
Princeton, NJ
USA

Mihaela Pop
University of Toronto
Toronto
Canada

Kawal Rhode
King's College
London
UK

Maxime Sermesant
Inria
Inria - Asclepios Team
Sophia-Antipolis
France

Alistair Young
Department of Anatomy Radiology, Grafton
Auckland University
Auckland
New Zealand

ISSN 0302-9743   ISSN 1611-3349   (electronic)
Lecture Notes in Computer Science
ISBN 978-3-319-28711-9   ISBN 978-3-319-28712-6   (eBook)
DOI 10.1007/978-3-319-28712-6

Library of Congress Control Number: 2015959912

LNCS Sublibrary: SL6 – Image Processing, Computer Vision, Pattern Recognition, and Graphics

This Springer imprint is published by SpringerNature
The registered company is Springer International Publishing AG Switzerland

Preface

Recently, there has been considerable progress in cardiac image analysis techniques, cardiac atlases, and computational models, which can integrate data on heart shape, function, and physiology from large-scale databases. Integrative models of cardiac function are important for understanding disease, evaluating treatment, and planning intervention. However, a significant clinical translation of these tools is constrained by the lack of complete and rigorous technical and clinical validation as well as by benchmarking of the developed tools. For doing so, common and available ground-truth data capturing generic knowledge on the healthy and pathological heart are required. This knowledge can be acquired through the building of statistical models of the heart. Several efforts are now established to provide Web-accessible structural and functional atlases of the normal and pathological heart for clinical work, research, and educational purposes. We believe all these approaches will only be effectively developed through collaborations across the full research scope of the imaging and modelling communities.

STACOM 2015 was held in conjunction with the MICCAI 2015 conference (Munich, Germany) and followed the past five editions: STACOM 2014 (Boston, USA), STACOM 2013 (Nagoya, Japan), STACOM 2012 (Nice, France), STACOM 2011 (Toronto, Canada), and STACOM 2010 (2010, Beijing, China). Our main goal is to provide a forum for the discussion of the latest developments in the areas of statistical atlases and computational imaging and modelling of the heart. The topics of the workshop include: cardiac image processing, atlas construction, statistical modelling of cardiac function across different patient populations, cardiac mapping, cardiac computational physiology, model customization, image-based modelling and image-guided interventional procedures, atlas-based functional analysis, ontological schemata for data and results, integrated functional and structural analyses, as well as the pre-clinical and clinical applicability of these methods. STACOM 2015 drew many submissions from around the world, with 23 papers finally accepted for presentation at the workshop. Beside regular contributions on various topics (e.g., state-of–the-art cardiac image analysis techniques, atlases, and computational models that integrate data on heart shape, function, and physiology from large-scale databases), additional efforts of this year's workshop focused on a statistical shape modelling challenge, briefly described here.

In addition to the papers presented, two keynote lectures were included in the program of STACOM 2015: Dr. Graham Wright of Sunnybrook Research Institute, University of Toronto (Canada), whose talk focused on "MRI for Guiding Ventricular Arrhythmia Management," and Dr. Mark Potse of Inria Bordeaux (France), who presented "Patient-Tailored Heart Models as a Diagnostic Modality."

Statistical shape modelling challenge: Statistical shape modeling is a powerful tool for visualizing and quantifying geometric and functional patterns of variation in the heart. Biologically, the heart exhibits great anatomical and functional variation making the encoding of these differences an interesting challenge in itself. After a myocardial infarction, the heart remodels in response to physiological challenges. The 2015

STACOM LV statistical shape modelling challenge was designed to test the hypothesis that a probabilistic model of the left ventricle can predict a patient's disease status. The goals of this challenge were to (a) establish a statistical shape model from the set of 3D shapes, and (b) develop an optimal classifier to distinguish between normal or diseased with myocardial infarct. Participants' methods could be supervised or unsupervised. Classification accuracy, specificity, and sensitivity measures were reported. The challenge provided additional insight into the methods that best describe left ventricular remodelling after myocardial infarction, attracting 11 participating groups, whose detailed methods and results are included in these proceedings. A collation journal paper including all results is planned in the near future. Preliminary results can be found on the workshop's website.

We hope that the results obtained by the challenge, together with all regular paper contributions, will act to accelerate progress in the important areas of heart function and structure analysis.

October 2015

Oscar Camara
Tommaso Mansi
Mihaela Pop
Kawal Rhode
Maxime Sermesant
Alistair Young

Organization

We would like to thank all organizers, additional reviewers, contributing authors, and sponsors for their time, effort, and financial support in making STACOM 2015 a successful event.

Workshop Chairs

Oscar Camara   Universitat Pompeu Fabra, Barcelona, Spain
Tommaso Mansi   Medical Imaging Technologies, Siemens Healthcare, Princeton, NJ, USA
Mihaela Pop   Medical Biophysics, University of Toronto, Sunnybrook Research Institute, Toronto, Canada
Kawal Rhode   King's College London, UK
Maxime Sermesant   Inria, Asclepios Project, Sophia Antipolis, France
Alistair Young   University of Auckland, New Zealand

Challenge Organizing Team

Statistical shape modelling challenge: Pau Medrano-Gracia, Avan Suinesiaputra, Alistair Young

Additional Reviewers

We would like to acknowledge the following reviewers who, in addition to the chairs and challenge organizers of the workshop, provided scientific feedback to the participants on the submitted papers: Constantine Butakoff, Nicholas Duchateau, Rocio Cabrera Lozoya, Sasa Grbic, Marie-Pierre Jolly, Antonio Porras Perez, Marc Michel Rohé, David Soto-Iglesias, Eduardo Soudah, Eranga Ukwatta, and Sergio Vera.

Sponsorship Liaison

Mihaela Pop   Medical Biophysics, University of Toronto, Sunnybrook Research Institute, Toronto, Canada

Submission/Publication Chairs

Mihaela Pop   Medical Biophysics, University of Toronto, Sunnybrook Research Institute, Toronto, Canada
Tommaso Mansi   Medical Imaging Technologies, Siemens Healthcare Princeton, NJ, USA

Webmaster

Pau Medrano-Gracia   University of Auckland, New Zealand

Workshop Website

http://capwebprd01.its.auckland.ac.nz/web/stacom2015

Sponsors

We are extremely grateful for the industrial funding support. The STACOM 2015 workshop received financial support from the following Silver and Elite Sponsors:

Imricor Medical Devices (http://www.imricor.com)

SciMedia Ltd. (http://www.scimedia.com/)

VisualSonics (http://visualsonics.com)

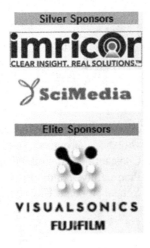

Contents

Shape Challenge Papers

Regular Papers

Automated Model-Based Left Ventricle Segmentation in Cardiac MR Images

Sharath Gopal$^{(\boxtimes)}$ and Demetri Terzopoulos

Computer Science Department, University of California, Los Angeles, USA
sharath@cs.ucla.edu

Abstract. We present a fully automated system for segmenting the Left Ventricle (LV) in cardiac MR images based on statistical and deformable models. A Project-Out Inverse Compositional Active Appearance Model of 3D LV shape produces segmentations that are refined using a unified statistical/deterministic deformable model. A new multi-scale detector, based on the Histogram of Oriented Gradients (HoG), produces initial estimates of LV position and scale in the MR volume. The performance of the HoG detector and the deformable-model-based segmentation components are evaluated on the 30 MICCAI Grand Challenge test images. The average F-measure for detector bounding box overlap is 0.89. The average F-measures for contour overlap are 0.80 (endo), 0.82 (epi), and 0.46 (myocardium).

1   Introduction

Left Ventricle (LV) segmentation in cardiac Magnetic Resonance (MR) images is a well-studied problem [14] that is clinically important in cardiac function analysis. Even though much research has been reported, full automation of accurate LV segmentation remains a challenge [16]. A fully automated system should be able to produce good LV shape reconstructions in the presence of moderate noise, intensity inhomogeneities, partial volume effects, patient motion misregistrations, and other cardiac MR imaging artifacts that can be detrimental to image analysis algorithms. In this work, we introduce a system that achieves the automation goal with as few assumptions as possible.

The key algorithms/components employed by our system and our main motivations for including them are as follows: A Project Out Inverse Compositional (POIC) Active Appearance Model (AAM) [11] underlies a model-based segmentation procedure and a unified statistical/deterministic deformable model refines the performance of the AAM. Due to the sensitivity of most optimization-based segmentation algorithms to model initialization, a good initial estimate of LV position and scale can help avoid convergence on sub-optimal local extrema. To provide good estimates, we propose a new multi-scale LV detector based on the Histogram of Oriented Gradients (HoG) [4].

© Springer International Publishing Switzerland 2016
O. Camara et al. (Eds.): STACOM 2015, LNCS 9534, pp. 3–12, 2016.
DOI: 10.1007/978-3-319-28712-6_1

2   Position and Scale Estimation

2.1   Multi-scale HoG Detector

Multi-scale HoG detectors are trained to estimate the position and scale of the LV in image slices from the base to the apex of the heart. The change in scale and appearance of the LV myocardium from the base to the apex is the main reason for having 3 different detectors (of 3 different scales) that are trained on basal, mid, and apical regions (Fig. 1).

Given a patient's image volume as a training case, it is first divided into 3 sets of slices from base to apex. For each of the 3 slice sets, a HoG feature vector (L_2 norm block normalization) is computed on every slice in that set and fed to a Support Vector Machine (SVM) classifier (linear, $C = 1$) [1] as positive training cases. Negative training cases are obtained by computing the HOG feature vector in the background of the slice in the respective set. The details of each HoG descriptor are given in Table 1.

Given a new patient's MR image slices, a sliding window detection algorithm is used to obtain a final bounding volume across the slices (Fig. 2). The algorithm's post-processing steps, listed in Procedure 1, deal with Non-Maximum Suppression (NMS), estimating the basal and apical slices, and finally choosing a combination of bounding boxes (BBs) that are better "aligned" along the LV longitudinal axis. The final output of this procedure is a set of BBs (each with its own size/scale), from the basal slice p to the apical slice q, which have been registered to remove any slice misregistration due to patient motion or breathing.

The volume bounded by the BBs provides an estimate of the position and scale of the LV in the images. The central line of the LV is the line through the

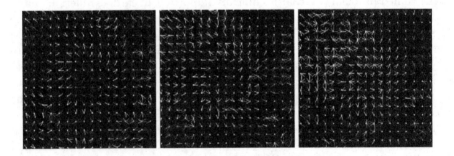

Fig. 1. HoGs visualized for Base (left), Mid (middle), and Apex (right) regions.

Table 1. HoG Feature Descriptors

Detector	Region	Box Size	Block Size	Cell Size	Block Stride	Bins
D_b	Base	80×80	10×10	5×5	5	9
D_m	Mid	60×60	6×6	3×3	3	9
D_a	Apex	42×42	6×6	3×3	3	9

Procedure 1. Left Ventricle Detector

Input: Image slices $1, 2, \ldots, N$

Output: Bounding box for each slice in range $p - q$, ($p < q$ and $1 \leq p$ and $q \leq N$), where p and q are the estimated basal and apical slices.

1 Compute SVM score masks $M_D = (m_1, m_2, \ldots, m_N)$ using sliding window detection for all detectors $D \in (D_b, D_m, D_a)$ across all N slices.

2 Compute a candidate BB set $C = (c_1, c_2, \ldots, c_N)$, where $c_i : i \in (1, 2, \ldots, N)$ is the candidate set of BBs for slice i, by performing NMS on M_{Db}, M_{Dm}, and M_{Da} score masks using an overlap threshold ϵ.

3 Set p to the smallest slice number such that candidate sets $c_1, c_2, \ldots, c_{p-1}$ are empty. Similarly, set q to the largest slice number such that candidate sets $c_{q+1}, c_{q+2}, \ldots, c_N$ are empty. If any set from c_p to c_q is empty, then fill them with averages of the BBs from neighboring slices.

4 Compute "scatter" scores for all possible combinations of BBs in the sets $c_p, c_{p+1}, \ldots, c_q$. For a given combination of BBs, $B_p, B_{p+1}, \ldots, B_q$, the scatter score is the sum of the 2 eigenvalues of the covariance matrix of the Gaussian fit to the 2D centers of the BBs. Select the combination with the least scatter score.

5 Register the slices p to q such that the centers for the final BBs line up along the longitudinal axis of the volume.

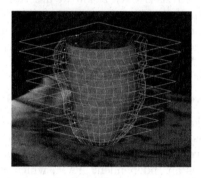

Fig. 2. Volume showing LV and detected bounding boxes.

center of each BB, from slice p to q, along the longitudinal axis. An approximate scale can be obtained by first producing a rough LV shape from the BBs, where 2 concentric circles (endo and epi) are placed within each BB at each slice in the range p–q. The epi contour is just the inscribed circle for the square BB. The endo contour has to be estimated from the quantity of pixels that belong to the blood pool. To do this in a principled way, we collect the intensity of all the pixels enclosed by the BBs across all slices, and fit a Gaussian Mixture Model (GMM) [3] with two modes. This GMM is subsequently used to classify the pixels as either blood pool or myocardium. The ratio of endo and epi contour radii is given by $\frac{r_{endo}}{r_{epi}} = \sqrt{\frac{A_{bp}}{A_{total}}}$, where A_{bp} is the number of pixels labelled as blood pool, and A_{total} is the total number of pixels inside the BB.

Using this approximate LV shape $\mathbf{t} \in R^n$ as the target shape, and given another LV shape $\mathbf{m} \in R^n$ that needs to be scaled by a factor k, we can minimize the following cost function:

$$\arg\min_{k} \|\mathbf{t} - k\mathbf{m}\|^2 \tag{1}$$

The minimizer is $k = \mathbf{m}^T\mathbf{t}/\|\mathbf{m}\|^2$. These initial estimates of position and scale are crucial for a segmentation system to be fully automated and less susceptible to suboptimal local minima.

3   Segmentation

Segmentation of the LV has been studied under two main types of methods based on the strength of the LV shape and appearance priors incorporated into the models [14]. On the one hand, deformable models [12] and pixel/image-based models [10] incorporate weak or no priors. On the other hand, statistical deformable models such as Active Shape Models (ASMs) and Active Appearance Models (AAMs) (see, e.g., [6,7,13,17]) include strongs priors learned via Principal Components Analysis (PCA). Below we describe the use of the Project Out Inverse Compositional (POIC) approach [11] to building a strong prior for the 3D shape and appearance of the LV in cardiac MR images. Subsequently, we describe a unified deformable model to further refine the estimates obtained from the AAM.

3.1   Project Out Inverse Compositional 3D AAM

AAMs learn linear models of shape and appearance variation. They are classified as Combined AAMs [2] or Independent AAMs [11] based, respectively, on whether or not they have a common set of parameters that control both shape and appearance. POIC is an Independent AAM, which we use to train linear models of shape and appearance on aligned (by Procrustes analysis) 3D shapes of LV, and shape-normalized appearance sampled cardiac MR image information within the 3D LV shape. PCA on such training data yields the following generative models of shape $\mathbf{s}$ and appearance $\mathbf{g}$:

$$\mathbf{s} = \bar{\mathbf{s}} + \mathbf{P}_s\mathbf{b}_s, \tag{2}$$

$$\mathbf{g} = \bar{\mathbf{g}} + \mathbf{P}_g\mathbf{b}_g. \tag{3}$$

The appearance model is trained by warping the training shapes to the base/mean shape $\bar{\mathbf{s}}$ using piecewise affine warping on the tetrahedral 3D tessellation.

Given a new set of images $I(\mathbf{x})$, the fitting process involves a Gauss-Newton minimization of the following non-linear cost function (error image), with respect to the parameters $\mathbf{b}_s$ and $\mathbf{b}_g$ (with reduced dimensions):

$$\|\bar{\mathbf{g}} + \mathbf{P}_g\mathbf{b}_g - I(\mathbf{W}(\mathbf{x}; \mathbf{b}_s))\|^2. \tag{4}$$

The ability to precompute the steepest descent images and the Hessian, makes POIC an efficient algorithm.

3.2   Unified Statistical/Deformable Model

The above AAM provides an estimate of the LV shape by linearly combining deformation modes with coefficients $\mathbf{b}_s$. Since this is a limited set of orthonormal modes, the actual solution might not be present in the subspace spanned by them. It can be challenging to obtain accurate segmentation estimates with just an AAM. Therefore, to further refine the segmentation, we employ a variant of the Unified Statistical/Deterministic deformable model [7].

The model's geometry consists of a 3D deformable "skin" superimposed on a reference PCA shape (as in the POIC (2)). The skin is composed of spring-edged cuboids (12 springs) that impose elastic/structural constraints on neighboring nodes present on the endo and epi surfaces. Applying Lagrangian dynamics, the model is then made dynamic with respect to its parameters, thus yielding the following (massless) equations of motion:

$$\mathbf{C}\dot{\mathbf{q}} + \mathbf{K}\mathbf{q} = \mathbf{f}_q, \tag{5}$$

where $\dot{\mathbf{q}}$ is the time derivative of the vector $\mathbf{q}$ of degrees of freedom (DOF) of the model, which includes the pose parameters, PCA parameters, and displacement parameters of the skin from the PCA reference shape, $\mathbf{C}\dot{\mathbf{q}}$ are damping forces, $\mathbf{K}\mathbf{q}$ are internal elastic forces, and $\mathbf{f}_q$ are image gradient-based external forces applied to the model. The stiffness matrix $\mathbf{K}$ can be assembled "element-wise" by using the spring element matrix $\begin{bmatrix} k & -k \\ -k & k \end{bmatrix}$, where k is the spring stiffness, which can be tuned to control the elasticity of the skin that deforms away from the reference shape under the influence of external forces. Finally, we initialize the PCA parameters in $\mathbf{q}$ to the values obtained from the POIC AAM fitting algorithm and explicitly time-integrate the above equations of motion under the influence of the image forces [7] that pull the skin towards nearby image intensity edges.

4   Results

The MICCAI Grand Challenge dataset [15], consisting of short-axis (SA) image slices for 15 training and 30 test cases, was used to train and test the HoG detector and the deformable-model-based segmentation components. Each of the 45 cases contains ground truth epicardial (epi) and endocardial (endo) contours for the end-diastolic (ED) phase, and just the endo contours for the end-systolic (ES) phase. We evaluate our system on the ED phase only. The C++ SVM implementation in LibSVM [1] was used for the HoG detector, and the MLPACK [3] implementation of GMM was used for labelling the BB pixels. We tested the three Linear SVMs ($C = 1$) of the HoG detector on the 30 cases by using an overlap threshold $\epsilon = 0.5$ for the NMS step. We used 8 shape modes for the

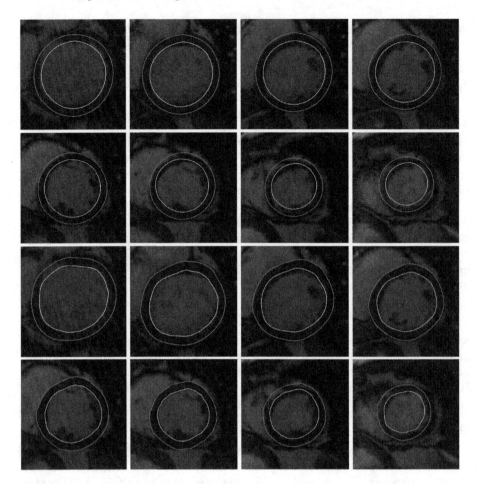

Fig. 3. Top 2 rows: POIC-AAM only. Bottom 2 rows: POIC-AAM + Refinement

POIC AAM and a spring constant $k = 0.5$ for the unified model. Except for assuming that the ED phase is known and the slices $1, 2, \ldots, N$ go from base to the apex, all components of the system are fully automated.

For each of these 30 cases, we report in Table 2 the precision and recall between the set of ground truth BB_{gt} and the estimated BB_{est} bounding boxes, which are calculated as $Recall = \frac{BB_{gt} \cap BB_{est}}{BB_{gt}}$ and $Precision = \frac{BB_{gt} \cap BB_{est}}{BB_{est}}$ (these are computed for the whole volume). For convenience, we also report in the table the F-measure (harmonic mean of precision and recall) for each case. Similarly, we evaluate the segmentation accuracy by computing the above 3 metrics with respect to overlap of areas for EPI (pixels inside the epi contour), ENDO (pixels inside the endo contour), and MYO (pixels in-between epi and endo contours).

The average F-measure for the detector BB overlap is 0.89. This shows that the detection system, as described in Procedure 1, is able to get good estimates

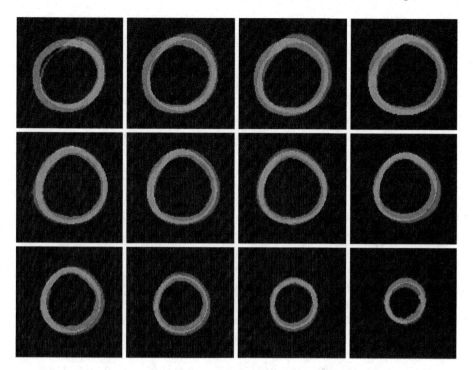

Fig. 4. Overlap of ground truth and estimated myocardial pixels (MYO) across slices. TP (yellow), FP (green), FN (red) and TN (black) (Color figure online).

of position and scale of the LV in the MR volume. The average F-measures for contour overlap are 0.80 for endo, 0.82 for epi, and 0.46 for myocardium. The potential refinement of the unified deformable model can be seen in Fig. 3 for the case HC-HF-I-05, where POIC-AAM only estimates are compared with those that have been further refined. We also show in Fig. 4, the myocardial overlap masks for case SC-HF-I-09 (with F-measure - 0.91 for endo, 0.93 for epi, 0.64 for myo). These images have been color coded to show the True Positive (TP), False Positive (FP), False Negative (FN) and True Negative (TN) myocardial labels obtained by overlaying the ground truth contours with the estimated contours. The myocardial F-measure is a good indicator of closeness between the estimated LV shape and the ground truth LV shape. It can be very challenging to get a high MYO F-measure due to the high degree of accuracy expected of a segmentation system on the test dataset.

To further investigate the performance, we measure the region-wise (base, mid, apex) contour overlap with respect to the ground truth contours (Recall). The average Recall for the base, mid and apex regions are as follows - endo (0.91, 0.89, 0.77), epi (0.90, 0.91, 0.81) and myo (0.50, 0.56, 0.43). These scores show that our automated system performs better at the base and mid LV regions when compared to the apex region. Dice coefficients and Average Perpendicular Distance

Table 2. Precision (P), Recall (R), and F-Measure (F)

ID	Case	Detector			ENDO			EPI			MYO		
		P	R	F	P	R	F	P	R	F	P	R	F
1	SC-HF-I-05	0.82	0.99	0.90	0.81	0.88	0.84	0.81	0.89	0.85	0.55	0.63	0.59
2	SC-HF-I-06	0.91	0.96	0.93	0.98	0.86	0.92	0.99	0.83	0.90	0.72	0.55	0.62
3	SC-HF-I-07	0.93	0.95	0.94	0.96	0.69	0.80	0.98	0.64	0.77	0.30	0.17	0.22
4	SC-HF-I-08	0.89	0.98	0.93	0.97	0.84	0.90	0.96	0.89	0.92	0.62	0.64	0.63
5	SC-HF-NI-07	0.87	0.94	0.91	0.97	0.82	0.89	0.95	0.89	0.92	0.56	0.62	0.59
6	SC-HF-NI-11	0.93	0.95	0.94	0.77	0.84	0.80	0.77	0.88	0.83	0.52	0.65	0.58
7	SC-HF-NI-31	0.88	0.98	0.93	0.73	0.93	0.82	0.70	0.98	0.82	0.32	0.53	0.40
8	SC-HF-NI-33	0.93	0.91	0.92	0.84	0.80	0.82	0.85	0.84	0.85	0.52	0.54	0.53
9	SC-HYP-06	0.89	0.95	0.92	0.79	0.82	0.81	0.81	0.78	0.80	0.53	0.46	0.49
10	SC-HYP-07	0.90	0.90	0.90	0.60	0.97	0.74	0.71	0.97	0.82	0.35	0.38	0.37
11	SC-HYP-08	0.83	0.88	0.86	0.59	0.86	0.70	0.71	0.77	0.74	0.54	0.41	0.47
12	SC-HYP-37	0.89	0.84	0.86	0.50	0.90	0.64	0.64	0.79	0.71	0.47	0.37	0.42
13	SC-N-05	0.88	0.89	0.89	0.89	0.83	0.86	0.96	0.78	0.86	0.62	0.41	0.49
14	SC-N-06	0.93	0.85	0.89	0.70	0.89	0.78	0.69	0.96	0.80	0.39	0.61	0.48
15	SC-N-07	0.77	0.98	0.86	0.66	0.99	0.79	0.64	0.99	0.78	0.19	0.31	0.24
16	SC-HF-I-09	0.87	0.98	0.93	0.96	0.87	0.91	0.93	0.93	0.93	0.58	0.72	0.64
17	SC-HF-I-10	0.85	0.98	0.91	0.91	0.89	0.90	0.88	0.92	0.90	0.54	0.65	0.59
18	SC-HF-I-11	0.84	0.97	0.90	0.93	0.90	0.91	0.85	0.95	0.90	0.50	0.74	0.59
19	SC-HF-I-12	0.85	0.94	0.90	0.95	0.84	0.89	0.97	0.83	0.89	0.67	0.53	0.59
20	SC-HF-NI-12	0.87	0.98	0.92	0.92	0.90	0.91	0.88	0.96	0.92	0.52	0.69	0.59
21	SC-HF-NI-13	0.75	0.93	0.83	0.69	0.86	0.77	0.65	0.94	0.77	0.19	0.38	0.25
22	SC-HF-NI-14	0.82	0.97	0.89	0.52	0.85	0.65	0.57	0.85	0.68	0.36	0.48	0.41
23	SC-HF-NI-15	0.62	0.98	0.76	0.39	0.79	0.52	0.41	0.85	0.55	0.17	0.37	0.23
24	SC-HYP-09	0.78	1.00	0.88	0.58	0.95	0.72	0.52	0.96	0.68	0.21	0.47	0.29
25	SC-HYP-10	0.94	0.91	0.93	1.00	0.70	0.82	1.00	0.71	0.83	0.36	0.26	0.30
26	SC-HYP-11	0.89	0.91	0.90	0.42	0.95	0.59	0.50	0.97	0.66	0.25	0.40	0.31
27	SC-HYP-12	0.83	0.93	0.88	1.00	0.72	0.84	0.99	0.78	0.87	0.46	0.42	0.44
28	SC-N-09	0.87	0.97	0.92	0.86	0.94	0.90	0.84	0.95	0.89	0.59	0.73	0.65
29	SC-N-10	0.74	0.93	0.82	0.61	0.92	0.74	0.81	0.91	0.86	0.52	0.41	0.45
30	SC-N-11	0.75	0.98	0.85	0.70	0.97	0.81	0.80	0.95	0.87	0.46	0.44	0.45
	Average	0.85	0.94	0.89	0.77	0.87	0.80	0.79	0.88	0.82	0.45	0.50	0.46

(APD) [15] were also measured for the test dataset. The dice coefficients were 0.87 and 0.89, and APD were 3.06 and 3.17 mm for endo and epi respectively. Results by other works (such as [5, 8, 9]) are either reported on private datasets or they include final averages for both ED and ES phases on the Grand Challenge dataset. Since our method has been applied only to the ED phase, an objective comparison of the final performance metrics will be hard.

Many semi-automated and manual LV segmentation systems and algorithms require some form of user interation, such as indicating the LV position in the image by clicking in the middle of the blood pool or by drawing a circle around it. As stated earlier, our main motivation for this work, is to build a system that is fully automated and produces 3D LV shape estimates from patient MR volumes with as few assumptions about the images as possible. Hence, we have focussed our efforts on trying to automatically reconstruct LV shapes that are close to the manually reconstructed LV shapes, without any clinical validation for now. The use of such a system in a clinical setting for LV mass, volumes and ejection fraction calculation requires automatically generated LV shapes for both ED and ES phases. As future work, we plan to build a similar system that performs temporal reconstruction of LV shapes, and also evaluate its accuracy and parameter sensitivity on a larger dataset, such as the consensus-based database of the Cardiac Atlas Project (CAP) [16].

5   Conclusion

We have presented a fully automated system to detect and segment the LV in cardiac MR images. The system employs a HoG-based multi-scale detector to obtain position and scale estimates of the LV in the MR volume. These estimates are crucial for optimization-based segmentation algorithms (POIC-AAM and the Unified Deformable Model), as they provide good initial model states that can aid in converging to the globally optimum solution. We tested the performance of our system on the 15 training and 30 test cases in the MICCAI Grand Challenge dataset, reporting precision, recall, and F-measures for the bounding box overlap and the contour overlap. The results show promise for the future use of such a system in a clinical setting for the reproducible reconstruction of LV shapes, without having to worry about any issues of inter- and intra-observer variability.

References

1. Chang, C.C., Lin, C.J.: LIBSVM: A library for support vector machines. ACM Trans. Intell. Syst. Technol. **2**, 27:1–27:27 (2011). http://www.csie.ntu.edu.tw/~cjlin/libsvm
2. Cootes, T.F., Edwards, G.J., Taylor, C.J.: Active appearance models. In: Burkhardt, H., Neumann, B. (eds.) ECCV 1998. LNCS, vol. 1407, pp. 484–498. Springer, Heidelberg (1998)
3. Curtin, R.R., Cline, J.R., Slagle, N.P., March, W.B., Ram, P., Mehta, N.A., Gray, A.G.: MLPACK: A scalable C++ machine learning library. J. Mach. Learn. Res. **14**, 801–805 (2013)
4. Dalal, N., Triggs, B.: Histograms of oriented gradients for human detection. In: IEEE Computer Society Conference on Computer Vision and Pattern Recognition (CVPR 2005), vol. 1, pp. 886–893. IEEE (2005)
5. Feng, C., Li, C., Zhao, D., Davatzikos, C., Litt, H.: Segmentation of the left ventricle using distance regularized two-layer level set approach. In: Mori, K., Sakuma, I., Sato, Y., Barillot, C., Navab, N. (eds.) MICCAI 2013, Part I. LNCS, vol. 8149, pp. 477–484. Springer, Heidelberg (2013)

6. Gopal, S., Otaki, Y., Arsanjani, R., Berman, D., Terzopoulos, D., Slomka, P.: Combining active appearance and deformable superquadric models for LV segmentation in cardiac MRI. In: SPIE Medical Imaging, p. 86690G. International Society for Optics and Photonics (2013)

7. Gopal, S., Terzopoulos, D.: A unified statistical/deterministic deformable model for LV segmentation in cardiac MRI. In: Camara, O., Mansi, T., Pop, M., Rhode, K., Sermesant, M., Young, A. (eds.) STACOM 2013. LNCS, vol. 8330, pp. 180–187. Springer, Heidelberg (2014)

8. Huang, S., Liu, J., Lee, L., Venkatesh, S., Teo, L., Au, C., Nowinski, W.: Segmentation of the left ventricle from cine MR images using a comprehensive approach. The MIDAS Journal - Cardiac MR Left Ventricle Segmentation Challenge (2009). http://hdl.handle.net/10380/3121

9. Lu, Y.L., Connelly, K.A., Dick, A.J., Wright, G.A., Radau, P.E.: Automatic functional analysis of left ventricle in cardiac cine MRI. Quant. Imaging Med. Surg. **3**(4), 200 (2013)

10. Lynch, M., Ghita, O., Whelan, P.F.: Automatic segmentation of the left ventricle cavity and myocardium in MRI data. Comput. Biol. Med. **36**(4), 389–407 (2006)

11. Matthews, I., Baker, S.: Active appearance models revisited. Int. J. Comput. Vis. **60**(2), 135–164 (2004)

12. McInerney, T., Terzopoulos, D.: A dynamic finite element surface model for segmentation and tracking in multidimensional medical images with application to cardiac 4d image analysis. Comput. Med. Imaging Graph. **19**(1), 69–83 (1995)

13. Mitchell, S.C., Bosch, J.G., Lelieveldt, B.P., van der Geest, R.J., Reiber, J.H., Sonka, M.: 3-D active appearance models: Segmentation of cardiac MR and ultrasound images. IEEE Trans. Med. Imaging **21**(9), 1167–1178 (2002)

14. Petitjean, C., Dacher, J.N.: A review of segmentation methods in short axis cardiac MR images. Med. Image Anal. **15**(2), 169–184 (2011)

15. Radau, P., Lu, Y., Connelly, K., Paul, G., Dick, A.J., Wright, G.A.: Evaluation framework for algorithms segmenting short axis cardiac MRI. The MIDAS Journal - Cardiac MR Left Ventricle Segmentation Challenge (2009). http://hdl.handle.net/10380/3070

16. Suinesiaputra, A., Cowan, B.R., Al-Agamy, A.O., Elattar, M.A., Ayache, N., Fahmy, A.S., Khalifa, A.M., Medrano-Gracia, P., Jolly, M.P., Kadish, A.H., et al.: A collaborative resource to build consensus for automated left ventricular segmentation of cardiac MR images. Med. Image Anal. **18**(1), 50–62 (2014)

17. Zhang, H., Wahle, A., Johnson, R.K., Scholz, T.D., Sonka, M.: 4-d cardiac MR image analysis: Left and right ventricular morphology and function. IEEE Trans. Med. Imag. **29**(2), 350–364 (2010)

Beyond the AHA 17-Segment Model: Motion-Driven Parcellation of the Left Ventricle

Wenjia Bai[1](✉), Devis Peressutti[2], Sarah Parisot[1], Ozan Oktay[1],
Martin Rajchl[1], Declan O'Regan[3], Stuart Cook[3,4], Andrew King[2],
and Daniel Rueckert[1]

[1] Biomedical Image Analysis Group, Department of Computing,
Imperial College London, London, UK
w.bai@imperial.ac.uk
[2] Division of Imaging Sciences and Biomedical Engineering,
King's College London, London, UK
[3] MRC Clinical Sciences Centre, Hammersmith Hospital,
Imperial College London, London, UK
[4] Duke-NUS Graduate Medical School, Singapore, Singapore

Abstract. A major challenge for cardiac motion analysis is the high-dimensionality of the motion data. Conventionally, the AHA model is used for dimensionality reduction, which divides the left ventricle into 17 segments using criteria based on anatomical structures. In this paper, a novel method is proposed to divide the left ventricle into homogeneous parcels in terms of motion trajectories. We demonstrate that the motion-driven parcellation has good reproducibility and use it for data reduction and motion description on a dataset of 1093 subjects. The resulting motion descriptor achieves high performance on two exemplar applications, namely gender and age predictions. The proposed method has the potential to be applied to groupwise motion analysis.

1 Introduction

The evaluation of cardiac function involves assessing not only the anatomy of the heart but also its motion [1,2]. Modern imaging modalities such as magnetic resonance (MR) and ultrasound (US) provide a convenient way for visualisation and analysis of cardiac motion. A major challenge for cardiac motion analysis is the high-dimensionality of the image data, both spatially and temporally. In order to reduce the dimensionality, the 17-segment model proposed by the American Heart Association (AHA) is conventionally used to divide the image data into regional segments using criteria based on anatomical structures [3].

For cardiac motion analysis, however, it is possible that certain regions with unique motion signatures, e.g. regions with scars or other pathologies, may not align with the pre-defined anatomical segments of the AHA model. In this work, we propose to parcellate the left ventricle (LV) into a number of segments such that each segment contains similar and consistent motion information. To the

© Springer International Publishing Switzerland 2016
O. Camara et al. (Eds.): STACOM 2015, LNCS 9534, pp. 13–20, 2016.
DOI: 10.1007/978-3-319-28712-6_2

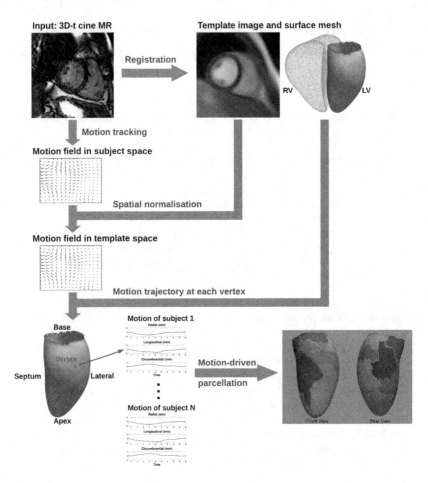

Fig. 1. The flowchart consists of motion tracking, spatial normalisation and motion-driven parcellation.

best of our knowledge, this is the first time that motion-driven parcellation is proposed for the heart, although a similar idea, functional parcellation, has become common for brain analysis [4]. Using a large dataset of cardiac MR images from 1093 subjects, we demonstrate that the parcellation has good reproducibility and can be used to reduce data dimensionality and be applied to cardiac motion analysis.

2 Methods

In this work, we are interested in the motion of the LV and parcellation is based on the motion tracking results for the LV. We employ a group-wise parcellation method, in which the motion fields of a large population are normalised onto a template surface mesh and then clustering is applied to the normalised motion feature vectors of the vertices. Figure 1 illustrates the flowchart of the method and we will explain each step in the following.

2.1 Data Description

The dataset used in this work consists of cardiac MR images of 1093 normal subjects (493 males, 600 females; age range 19–75 yr, mean 40.1 yr). Cardiac MR was performed on a 1.5T Philips Achieva system (Best, Netherlands) using the 3D cine balanced steady-state free precession (b-SSFP) sequence. The voxel spacing is 1.25×1.25×2 mm. Cine MR images are used here for cardiac motion analysis, which consists of 20 time frames across a cardiac cycle with the 0-th frame representing the end-diastolic (ED) frame. Other imaging modalities such as tagged MR or ultrasound may also be used, which can capture the motion of the heart at a different spatio-temporal resolution and with different quality.

2.2 Motion Tracking

Motion tracking is performed for each subject using a 4D spatio-temporal B-spline image registration method with a sparseness regularisation term [5]. The motion field estimate is represented in the subject space by a displacement vector at each voxel and at each time frame t, which measures the displacement from the 0-th frame to the t-th frame.

2.3 Spatial Normalisation

Parcellation is performed in a template image space, as shown at the top-right corner of Fig. 1. To represent the motion fields of all the subjects in the template space, the subject images are aligned to the template image by non-rigid B-spline image registration [6]. Using the transformation between the template space and subject space, the motion field of each subject is transported to the template space. Let $\mathbf{x}' = T(\mathbf{x})$ denote the transformation from template to subject, where $\mathbf{x}$ and $\mathbf{x}'$ are respectively the coordinates in the template space and in the subject space. By considering the spatial transformation as a change of coordinates [7], we have,

$$\mathbf{d}(\mathbf{x}, t) = \mathbf{J}_{T^{-1}}(\mathbf{x}') \cdot \mathbf{d}'(\mathbf{x}', t) \tag{1}$$

where $\mathbf{d}'$ denotes the displacement in the subject space, $\mathbf{d}$ denotes the corresponding displacement in the template space and $\mathbf{J}_{T^{-1}}(\mathbf{x}') \equiv \frac{d\mathbf{x}}{d\mathbf{x}'}$ denotes the Jacobian matrix of the inverse transformation.

2.4 Motion-Driven Parcellation

Let M denote the number of vertices on the template surface mesh (8528 vertices in our case), N denote the number of subjects and F denote the dimension of the motion trajectory. The motion trajectory at a vertex is defined as the concatenation of the radial, longitudinal and circumferential displacements of all the time frames across the cardiac cycle. Then at each vertex, we concatenate the motion trajectory of all the subjects, resulting in a feature vector of dimension $n = NF$. Parcellation can be regarded as clustering of the M vertices into K groups such that the vertices in each group display similar group-wise motion trajectory. It produces a reduced representation of the input data.

A number of approaches have been proposed for clustering, such as K-means, Ward's algorithm [8], EM algorithm which models the clusters as a mixture of Gaussians or other distributions [9] and graph partitioning [10]. We use the Ward's algorithm which has been shown to perform with good reproducibility in [11].

Ward's algorithm starts by considering each vertex as a cluster [8]. Then at each step, it merges the two closest clusters. It defines the loss function as the within-cluster variance and the two clusters which lead to the minimal increase of the loss function are selected for merging,

$$(c_1, c_2) = \arg\min_{c_1, c_2} \sum_{i \in c_1 \cup c_2} ||\mathbf{y}_i - \bar{\mathbf{y}}_{c_1 \cup c_2}||^2 - \left(\sum_{i \in c_1} ||\mathbf{y}_i - \bar{\mathbf{y}}_{c_1}||^2 + \sum_{i \in c_2} ||\mathbf{y}_i - \bar{\mathbf{y}}_{c_2}||^2 \right)$$

(2)

where c_1 and c_2 denote the clusters to be merged, $\mathbf{y}_i$ denotes a data point in the cluster and $\bar{\mathbf{y}}$ denotes the cluster mean.

The feature vector at each vertex is of n dimension. To reduce the computational cost of clustering, we reduce the dimension of the feature vector using PCA. We keep the first few principal components which account for 95 % of the data variance and thus reduce the feature vector dimension to 36. Ward's clustering is applied to the data after dimensionality reduction.

2.5 Reproducibility Index

To evaluate the reproducibility of the clustering or the parcellation, we use the Rand index as in work [11], which measures the agreements between two clustering results [12]. For M vertices, the total number of vertex pairs is $\binom{M}{2}$. Let a denote the number of vertex pairs that are placed in the same class in clustering 1 and also in the same class in clustering 2, b denote the number of vertex pairs that are placed in different classes in clustering 1 and also in different classes in clustering 2. The Rand index is defined as $R = (a+b)/\binom{M}{2}$. It is a value between 0 and 1, with 0 indicating that two clusterings do not agree with each other at all and 1 indicating that two clusterings are the same.

3 Experiments and Results

3.1 Visualisation

We empirically set the number of clusters for Ward's clustering to 17 to be comparable with the AHA 17-segment model. Figure 2 compares the AHA 17-segment model with the 17-segment model produced by motion-driven parcellation, which we name as "functional 17-segment model" for short. The AHA

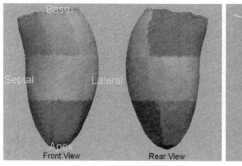 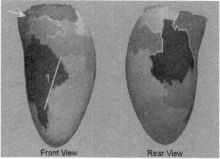

(a) AHA 17-segment model   (b) Functional 17-segment model

Fig. 2. Comparison of the anatomical segment model with the functional segment model.

model, Fig. 2(a), distributes 35 % of the volume to the basal part (6 segments), 35 % to the mid-ventricular part (6 segments), 30 % to the apical part (4 segments) and 5 % to the apex [3]. The functional 17-segment model does not follow the empirical definition for the volume percentage, but instead it creates segments which have homogeneous motion trajectories. There are several interesting findings in the functionally parcellated model, as shown in Fig. 2(b). First, the segments are not of equal size. Those at the basal part (pointed by the arrow) are relatively small, which hints that the variance of motion is large at this part so the parcellation needs to be dense. Second, the septal wall (left of line 1) is separated from the other parts of the wall (right of line 1), which is physiologically reasonable, because the motion of the septal wall is restricted by its connection with the right ventricle while the other parts are more free.

3.2 Reproducibility

We evaluate the reproducibility of the parcellation by comparing the clustering results on two subsets. We randomly select 500 subjects as the first set and 500 subjects as the second set and the two sets are mutually exclusive. Motion-driven parcellation is performed on both sets and the clustering results are compared visually and quantitatively. As Fig. 3 shows, the septal wall (left of line 1) is consistently separated from the lateral wall (right of line 1) on both subsets. The basal part (above line 2) is consistently separated from the mid-ventricular part (below line 2). The separations at line 3 and line 4 are also consistent. These separating lines and regions are also noticeable on the parcellation based on the full dataset, Fig. 2(b).

To quantitatively evaluate the reproducibility of parcellation, we repeat the random subset division for 10 times and measure the Rand index between the two parcellations. The mean Rand index is 0.922 ± 0.006. This means that for 92.2 % of the vertex pairs, the two parcellations agree on whether or not they belong to the same parcel.

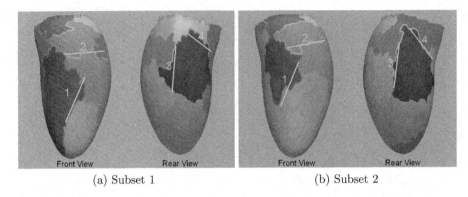

(a) Subset 1   (b) Subset 2

Fig. 3. The parcellation results based on two mutually exclusive subsets, each containing 500 subjects. The colour codes of the two parcellations are not exactly the same, because the cluster IDs given by the Ward's algorithm can be different in two runs. Please refer to the paragraph for the explanation of the lines (Color figure online).

Table 1. Gender and age prediction performance using the motion descriptors with different number of parcels and with the AHA 17-segment model.

	Gender Accuracy	Age Correlation
7 parcels	87.4 %	0.823
17 parcels	88.0 %	0.830
27 parcels	**89.0 %**	0.831
37 parcels	88.6 %	**0.834**
AHA	88.9 %	0.827

3.3   Application: Classification

Parcellation is often used for dimensionality reduction and it has a wide range of potential applications. In this study, we use it to extract a motion descriptor for cardiac motion analysis. We compute the mean motion trajectory for each parcel and concatenate them to form a motion descriptor of the left ventricle. We demonstrate the ability of the motion descriptor using two exemplar classification tasks, gender classification and age prediction. For comparison, we test the performance when different numbers of clusters are used in parcellation and when the AHA 17-segment model is used for computing the motion descriptor.

We performed 10-fold cross-validation on the set of 1093 subjects. Given the motion descriptor as input, SVM classifiers with RBF kernels were trained on the training set and then applied to the testing set to predict the gender and age of a given subject. The prediction accuracy for gender and the correlation coefficient between predicted age and real age are evaluated. The results are reported in Table 1 and plotted in Fig. 4. It shows that using the parcellation-based motion descriptor, we can achieve high accuracy for both gender and age prediction. For gender prediction, motion-driven parcellation using 27 segments

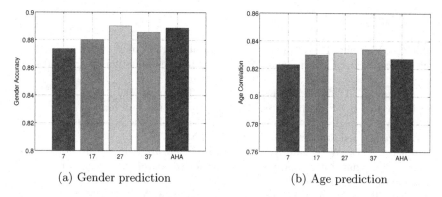

(a) Gender prediction   (b) Age prediction

Fig. 4. Gender and age prediction performance using the motion descriptors with different number of parcels (7, 17, 27 or 37 parcels) and with the AHA 17-segment model.

achieves slightly better performance than the AHA model ($p > 0.01$). For age prediction, motion-driven parcellation using 17, 27 or 37 parcels perform better than the AHA model ($p < 0.01$). In addition, using a small number of parcels such as 7 only slightly sacrifices the performance. The reason is that gender and age affects the cardiac motion globally and therefore a small number of parcels can also encode the information.

4 Conclusions

To conclude, a novel method is proposed for cardiac motion analysis, which parcellates the left ventricle based on motion information instead of using pre-defined anatomical structure. Although each individual component of the method (registration, transport and clustering) may not be novel in itself, they are combined to form a novel way to investigate cardiac motion. It can be used for visualising regional clustering of motion and for reducing high-dimensional motion data. As an exploratory step in this direction, we use the displacement trajectory to represent cardiac motion, but other representation such as velocity, strain or electroanatomical recording can be explored in future in this framework.

In the work, our data are all healthy subjects and therefore we only demonstrate the motion descriptor on two exemplar classifications, gender and age predictions. These two factors affect motion globally and may not be the best examples for demonstrating a regional descriptor. However, the proposed method has the potential to be extended to other applications, where regional descriptors are more important. For example, it can be used for groupwise motion analysis in which two groups of subjects present different local motion patterns.

A limitation of the proposed method is that it may be more suited to group analysis instead of case studies. A direction of future work is to include patients data with similar pathologies into our dataset and to perform motion analysis and comparison between the healthy and the patients.

References

1. Mor-Avi, V., Lang, R.M., Badano, L.P., Belohlavek, M., et al.: Current and evolving echocardiographic techniques for the quantitative evaluation of cardiac mechanics. Eur. J. Echocardiogr. **12**(3), 167–205 (2011)
2. Suinesiaputra, A., Frangi, A.F., Kaandorp, T., Lamb, H.J., Bax, J.J., Reiber, J., Lelieveldt, B.P.F.: Automated detection of regional wall motion abnormalities based on a statistical model applied to multislice short-axis cardiac MR images. IEEE Trans. Med. Imaging **28**(4), 595–607 (2009)
3. Cerqueira, M.D., Weissman, N.J., Dilsizian, V., Jacobs, A.K., et al.: Standardized myocardial segmentation and nomenclature for tomographic imaging of the heart. Circulation **105**(4), 539–542 (2002)
4. Yeo, B.T.T., Krienen, F.M., Sepulcre, J., Sabuncu, M.R., Lashkari, D., et al.: The organization of the human cerebral cortex estimated by intrinsic functional connectivity. J. Neurophysiol. **106**(3), 1125–1165 (2011)
5. Shi, W., Jantsch, M., Aljabar, P., Pizarro, L., Bai, W., Wang, H., O'Regan, D., Zhuang, X., Rueckert, D.: Temporal sparse free-form deformations. Med. Image Anal. **17**(7), 779–789 (2013)
6. Rueckert, D., Sonoda, L.I., Hayes, C., Hill, D.L.G., Leach, M.O., Hawkes, D.J.: Nonrigid registration using free-form deformations: application to breast MR images. IEEE Trans. Med. Imag. **18**(8), 712–721 (1999)
7. Duchateau, N., De Craene, M., Piella, G., Silva, E., Doltra, A., Sitges, M., Bijnens, B.H., Frangi, A.F.: A spatiotemporal statistical atlas of motion for the quantification of abnormal myocardial tissue velocities. Med. Image Anal. **15**(3), 316–328 (2011)
8. Ward, J.H.: Hierarchical grouping to optimize an objective function. J. Am. Stat. Assoc. **58**(301), 236–244 (1963)
9. Kulis, B., Jordan, M.I.: Revisiting k-means: New algorithms via Bayesian nonparametrics. In: ICML, pp. 513–520 (2012)
10. Shi, J., Malik, J.: Normalized cuts and image segmentation. IEEE Trans. Pattern Anal. Mach. Intell. **22**(8), 888–905 (2000)
11. Thirion, B., Varoquaux, G., Dohmatob, E., Poline, J.B.: Which fMRI clustering gives good brain parcellations? Front. Neurosci. **8**, 13 (2014)
12. Hubert, L., Arabie, P.: Comparing partitions. J. Classif. **2**(1), 193–218 (1985)

A Non-parametric Statistical Shape Model for Assessment of the Surgically Repaired Aortic Arch in Coarctation of the Aorta: How Normal Is Abnormal?

Jan L. Bruse[1]([✉]), Kristin McLeod[2], Giovanni Biglino[1],
Hopewell N. Ntsinjana[1], Claudio Capelli[1], Tain-Yen Hsia[1,4],
Maxime Sermesant[3], Xavier Pennec[3],
Andrew M. Taylor[1,4], and Silvia Schievano[1,4]

[1] Centre for Cardiovascular Imaging, Institute of Cardiovascular Science
and Cardiorespiratory Unit, University College London,
Great Ormond Street Hospital for Children, London, UK
jan.bruse.12@ucl.ac.uk
[2] Cardiac Modelling Department, Simula Research Laboratory, Oslo, Norway
[3] Inria, Asclepios Project, Sophia Antipolis, France
[4] Modeling of Congenital Hearts Alliance (MOCHA) Group, London, UK

Abstract. Coarctation of the Aorta (CoA) is a cardiac defect that requires surgical intervention aiming to restore an unobstructed aortic arch shape. Many patients suffer from complications post-repair, which are commonly associated with arch shape abnormalities. Determining the degree of shape abnormality could improve risk stratification in recommended screening procedures. Yet, traditional morphometry struggles to capture the highly complex arch geometries. Therefore, we use a non-parametric Statistical Shape Model based on mathematical currents to fully account for 3D global and regional shape features. By computing a template aorta of a population of healthy subjects and analysing its transformations towards CoA arch shape models using Partial Least Squares regression techniques, we derived a shape vector as a measure of subject-specific shape abnormality. Results were compared to a shape ranking by clinical experts. Our study suggests Statistical Shape Modelling to be a promising diagnostic tool for improved screening of complex cardiac defects.

Keywords: Non-parametric statistical shape model · Mathematical currents · Partial least square regression · Coarctation of the aorta · Aortic arch

1 Introduction

Coarctation of the Aorta (CoA) has an incidence of around 1 in 2500 live births [1]. Defined as a discrete or long obstruction of the aortic arch at the transverse,

© Springer International Publishing Switzerland 2016
O. Camara et al. (Eds.): STACOM 2015, LNCS 9534, pp. 21–29, 2016.
DOI: 10.1007/978-3-319-28712-6_3

isthmus or descending aorta level, it requires surgery to restore an unobstructed arch shape. Although survival rates have improved over the last decades, many patients suffer from late complications post-aortic arch repair such as hypertension, which have been associated with shape abnormalities of the arch [2]. Recent studies therefore suggest long-term follow-up and regular screening via cardiac imaging [1]. Being able to quantify the degree of shape abnormality could be beneficial for such screening procedures as it assists in identifying highly abnormal cases that are potentially associated with a higher risk profile. Yet, in clinical practice, aortic arch shape is commonly assessed via conventional 2D morphometry – without fully exploiting the shape information provided by current imaging technology. A multitude of geometric shape parameters is necessary to describe the complex tortuous arches, and landmarks for measuring deviations between shapes are difficult to select. Apart from the inherent measurement bias, such data are rather tedious to interpret and analyse. Statistical Shape Models (SSM) provide a visual, thus intuitively comprehensible tool to assess the entire 3D anatomy of a population of shapes [3]. Furthermore, the introduction of mathematical currents of surfaces as non-parametric anatomical shape descriptors [4] circumvents the process of landmarking and allows a robust and efficient analysis of shape features in complex shape populations.

In this paper, we aimed to build a SSM based on 3D surface models of aortic arches reconstructed from cardiovascular magnetic resonance (CMR) data in order to quantify the degree of shape abnormality of CoA arch shapes compared to the healthy aorta. The method is based on the *forward approach*, whereby transformations of an ideal unbiased template shape towards each subject shape within the population encode all global and regional 3D shape information [5,6]. We hypothesised that by analysing how a template shape of a healthy (not surgically altered) arch transforms towards each CoA arch shape, a shape vector as a subject-specific measure of abnormality can be derived. The shape vector essentially condenses 3D shape features down to a single number for each CoA patient, which allows a ranking of CoA shapes according to their overall shape deviation from the template. This was compared with an expert ranking of shape abnormality performed by three clinical experts, in order to explore to which degree the shape vector reflects the experts' opinion. Furthermore, we analyse associations between the expert ranking and conventional 2D shape descriptors that are commonly used in clinical practice.

2   Methods

2.1   Patient Population

This is a retrospective study based on a population of 20 healthy Control subjects and 20 age- and body surface area (BSA)-matched patients post-aortic arch repair (CoA) [7]. BSA was calculated using DuBois's formula [8]. Average age was 15.2 ± 2.0 years (mean ± standard deviation) for the Control and 16.5 ± 3.1 years for the CoA group. CoA patients had surgical arch repair four days to five years after birth. Control subjects did not have any intervention on the aortic arch and were considered "normal" in terms of shape.

2.2 Image Acquisition, Segmentation and Pre-processing of the Surface Models

40 aortas were segmented manually (Mimics, Leuven, Belgium) from whole-heart images acquired during mid-diastolic rest via CMR examination (1.5T Avanto MR scanner, Siemens Medical Solutions, Erlangen, Germany; 3D balanced steady-state free precession sequence; voxel size 1.5×1.5×1.5 mm) [7]. Segmented models were cut at the aortic root and at the level of the diaphragm. Coronary arteries and head and neck vessels were removed. Surface models of the arches were meshed with 0.75 triangular cells/mm^2 and smoothed with a pass-band filter (VMTK, The Vascular Modeling Toolkit, Bergamo, Italy [9]). Prior to computing the template shape, Control arches were rigidly aligned to an initial reference subject from the Control population using an Iterative Closest Point algorithm in VMTK [10]. As conventional 2D morphometric shape descriptors, the coarctation index ($CoAi$) and the ratio of arch height A to width T, A/T were measured on CMR images as proposed by Tan [11] and Ou [2], respectively.

2.3 Expert Assessment of the Aortic Arch Shapes

Three clinical experts (radiologist, cardiac surgeon and cardiologist; each with >10 years of experience) qualitatively ranked the CoA shapes according to their distance from a normal arch shape ($1 = close$; $2 = fairly\ close$; $3 = mid\text{-}range$; $4 = far\ away$; $5 = very\ far\ away$ from normal). Control arch shapes were accessible for comparison. The experts assessed the arches' surface models, merely using a 3D viewer[1], without knowing the patients' clinical history or results of the shape analysis.

2.4 Computation of the Control Template and its Transformations Towards CoA Subject Shapes

The template (i.e. mean shape) of the Control group was computed with the *exoshape* code framework as proposed by Durrleman [6] and introduced to cardiac research by Mansi [5], using mathematical currents [4] as non-parametric shape descriptors. Based on a *forward approach* [6], the template $\overline{T}$ and its transformations φ^i towards each subject shape T^i are computed simultaneously using an alternate two-step algorithm, minimising the distance between the deformed template $\varphi^i(\overline{T})$ and T^i in the vector space of currents. The latter is generated by two Gaussian kernels: K_W for the shape representations and K_V for the transformations φ. The associated kernel widths λ_W and λ_V are defined as the *resolution* of the currents representation and the *stiffness* of the deformations,

---

[1] 3D viewable models of the arches available under http://www.ucl.ac.uk/cardiac-engineering/research/library-of-3d-anatomies/congenital_defects/coarctations.

respectively [5]. In order to find an adequate set of λ parameters, an initial template of the Control group $\overline{T}_{Control,initial}$ was computed using starting values of $\lambda_{W,initial} = 15$ mm and $\lambda_{V,initial} = 47$ mm. As our analyis is based on analysing transformations that match the Control template with CoA shapes, the final set of λ parameters was obtained by matching $\overline{T}_{Control,initial}$ with a specific target shape from the CoA group $T^i_{CoA,Target}$, while incrementally decreasing $\lambda_{W,initial}$ and $\lambda_{V,initial}$ until the registration error between the deformed source shape $\varphi^i(\overline{T}_{Control,initial})$ and $T^i_{CoA,Target}$ was reduced by at least 80 %. Being one of the arch models that posed the most challenging shape features to be captured, the CoA subject with the smallest surface area was chosen as $T^i_{CoA,Target}$ (CoA3). Prior to the λ estimation, $T^i_{CoA,Target}$ was rigidly registered to $\overline{T}_{Control,initial}$. Based on this approach, $\lambda_W = 9$ mm and $\lambda_V = 44$ mm were found to allow sufficient matching of $\overline{T}_{Control,initial}$ with $T^i_{CoA,Target}$ and all other subjects, and were used to compute the final Control template $\overline{T}_{Control,final}$. After rigidly registering all CoA arch shapes to $\overline{T}_{Control,final}$, the transformations φ^i of $\overline{T}_{Control,final}$ towards each of the CoA subject shapes were computed using the same set of λ parameters. $\overline{T}_{Control,final}$ was validated using 10-fold cross-validation [5]. Further, gross geometric parameters of $\overline{T}_{Control,final}$ (volume V, surface area A_{surf}, centreline length L_{CL} and median diameter along the centreline D_{med}) were compared to the respective mean values of the Control population.

2.5 Analysing the Transformations Using Partial Least Squares Regression

The transformations φ, encoding all shape features present in the population, are parametrised by moment vectors β, which deform $\overline{T}_{Control,final}$ towards each subject shape in the space of currents [5]. The moment vectors β, obtained from transforming $\overline{T}_{Control,final}$ towards all Control and CoA shapes, constituted the input (predictors) for a Partial Least Squares regression (PLS). PLS extracts shape modes that maximise the covariance of predictors X and response Y [12]. To first extract shape features predominantly related to size differences between subjects, an initial *PLS I* was performed with all moment vectors β as predictors X_I and BSA of the subjects as response Y_I. A second *PLS II* was performed on the predictor residuals of *PLS I*, $X_{I,resid}$ using the grouping parameter Y_{II} ($0 = Control$; $1 = CoA$) as response. Residuals were defined as $X_{I,resid} = X_I - XS_{BSA} \times XL_{BSA}$ with XS_{BSA} being the predictor scores and XL_{BSA} being the predictor loadings of *PLS I*. Thereby, dominant shape features related to size differences were removed prior to extracting the shape mode most related to the grouping parameter. Shape modes were computed using the SIMPLS algorithm in Matlab (The MathWorks, Natick, MA) and the mean squared prediction error (MSEP) was estimated using 10-fold cross-validation. Only one *PLS I* and *PLS II* mode was retained as MSEP was not substantially decreased by adding more modes. By projecting each subject shape transformation onto the final shape mode *PLS II*, we derived the shape vector S [5]. It contains subject-specific weights, describing how much the template has to be deformed along the extracted mode in order to match template and subject shape as accurately as possible.

We hypothesised that the weights associated with the final shape mode yield a notion of how distant a specific subject shape is from the Control template shape – with large positive values representing subjects "far away" and small, negative numbers representing subjects "close" to the normal arch shape.

Correlations between the subject-specific entries of S, $CoAi$, A/T and the expert scores were assessed using Kendall's τ for non-parametric and ranked data. Non-parametric Mann-Whitney-U Test was applied to analyse shape vector differences between the two groups. Consistency between the expert ranking was assessed using the Intraclass Correlation Coefficient (ICC) assuming a 2-way mixed effects model. The significance level was set to p<.05. Statistical tests were carried out in SPSS (IBM SPSS Statistics, Chicago, IL).

3 Experiments and Results

3.1 Control Template

The final Control template showed a smooth, rounded aortic arch with a subtle tapering from ascending to descending aorta (Fig. 1a,b,c). Gross geometric parameters were close to their respective means measured on the entire Control population. Deviations ranged from 0.3 % (volume) to 1.94 % (median diameter), resulting in an overall average deviation of 1.02 %. Cross-validation revealed that the template shape was not substantially influenced by removing specific subjects from the analysis (Fig. 1d). Average surface distances between the full dataset shape and the reduced dataset shapes ranged from 0.14 to 1.22 mm.

side view	front view	top view	cross-validation

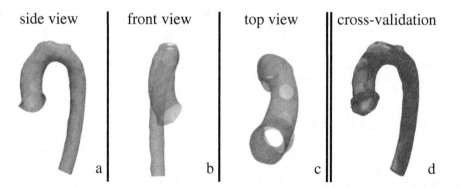

| a | b | c | d |

Fig. 1. Computed template shape of the Control population (a,b,c) and overlay of cross-validated template shapes based on reduced datasets (d, dark blue) (Color figure online)

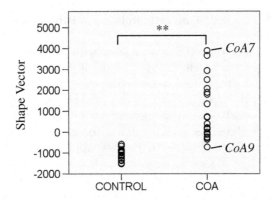

Fig. 2. PLS II shape vector results for Control and CoA group. Extreme subjects marked

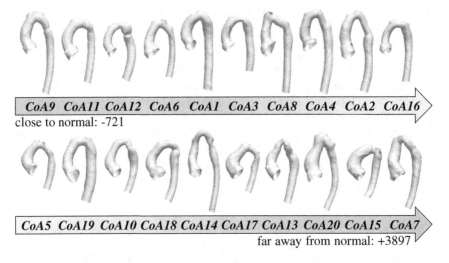

Fig. 3. Computed ranking of CoA arch shapes from *normal* (low shape vector values) to *abnormal* (high shape vector values)

3.2 PLS Regression Results

PLS I extracted shape features most related to BSA such as overall differences in size between subjects. The model yielded a good fit of BSA based on the derived *PLS I* shape mode ($r = 0.70$; $p \leq .001$), which accounted for 18 % of shape variability. *PLS II* derived shape features most related to either the Control or the CoA group. The *PLS II* shape mode accounted for 21 % of the remaining shape variability.

The *PLS II* shape mode weights of Control subjects clustered closer together (-1036 ± 252; mean $\pm$ standard deviation), whereas weights derived for CoA subjects showed a larger spread (1036 ± 1396), related to more shape variability

Table 1. Correlations between expert ranking and conventional 2D shape descriptors

	Expert 1		Expert 2		Expert 3		Average	
	τ	Significance	τ	Significance	τ	Significance	τ	Significance
CoAi	−0.11	p = .520	−0.04	p = .838	−0.22	p = .222	−0.11	p = .533
A/T	0.18	p = .919	0.13	p = .453	0.02	p = .892	0.06	p = .718

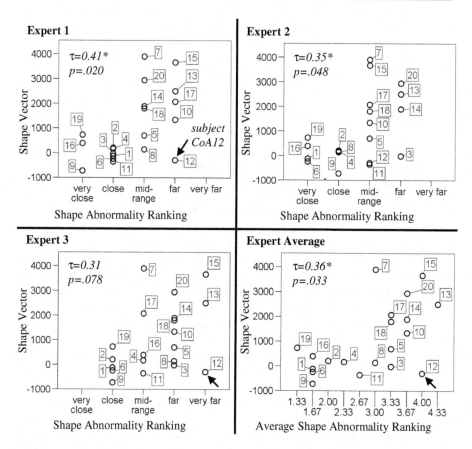

Fig. 4. Correlations between expert ranking of shape abnormality and computed shape vector values: Apart from the mid-range, trends were captured well. Outlier marked

within the CoA group. The distribution of shape vector values was significantly different (p≤.001) between the two groups (Fig. 2). Control subjects were associated with weight values between −1521 and −581; CoA subjects ranged from −721 to +3897 (Fig. 3).

3.3   Comparison of Expert Ranking with Shape Model Results

Qualitative shape rankings were consistent for experts 1 and 2 (mean scores 2.65 and 2.60), while expert 3 on average ranked CoA shapes farther away from normal (mean score 3.40). However, all experts applied a similar range of scores (all standard deviations 1.04).

Average ranking was reliable with ICC $= 0.88$ (p $\leq .001$). Conventional shape descriptors $CoAi$ and A/T did not correlate with the experts' ranking (Table 1). Expert shape scores correlated well with the computed shape vector for experts 1 and 2, and less for expert 3 (Fig. 4). Average expert ranking however, showed good correlation (Kendall's $\tau = 0.36$, p $= .033$).

4   Discussion and Conclusion

In this paper we analysed the transformations of a "normal" template aorta shape towards surgically repaired CoA arch shapes via PLS, in order to derive a subject-specific measure of shape abnormality. Particularly in the extreme cases of CoA shapes being either close or far away from normal, the derived shape vector reflected the expert ranking well. In the mid-range however, our method struggled to differentiate expert scores sufficiently. In particular one subject (CoA12) contributed to weak correlations between shape vector and expert rankings (Fig. 4). With a severe transverse narrowing and a highly localised indentation, subject CoA12 presents sophisticated shape features to be captured (Fig. 3). A decrease of the λ parameters might improve the method's accuracy – though at the expense of computation time. The main limitation of our study is the small sample size for both groups, which impeded applying more elaborate statistics and which should be addressed in future studies.

Interestingly though, the derived shape vector seemed to reflect the experts' shape assessment better than conventional 2D arch shape descriptors as typically used in clinical practice. This suggests Statistical Shape Modelling on 3D shapes to account for more relevant shape information and thus to come closer to an intuitive human shape assessment. Ultimately, applying Statistical Shape Models for clinical decision support could lead to more robust, efficient and objective diagnosis and risk stratification strategies in complex cardiac disease.

Acknowledgments. This study is independent research by the National Institute for Health Research Biomedical Research Centre Funding Scheme. The views expressed in this publication are those of the author(s) and not necessarily those of the NHS, the National Institute for Health Research or the Department of Health. The authors gratefully acknowledge support from Fondation Leducq, FP7 Integrated Project MD-Paedigree, National Institute of Health Research, Commonwealth Scholarship Comission and Heart Research UK.

References

1. Brown, M.L., Burkhart, H.M., Connolly, H.M., Dearani, J.A., Cetta, F., Li, Z., Oliver, W.C., Warnes, C.A., Schaff, H.V.: Coarctation of the aorta: lifelong surveillance is mandatory following surgical repair. J. Am. Coll. Cardiol. **62**, 1020–1025 (2013)
2. Ou, P., Bonnet, D., Auriacombe, L., Pedroni, E., Balleux, F., Sidi, D., Mousseaux, E.: Late systemic hypertension and aortic arch geometry after successful repair of coarctation of the aorta. Eur. Heart J. **25**, 1853–1859 (2004)
3. Young, A.A., Frangi, A.F.: Computational cardiac atlases: from patient to population and back. Exp Physiol. **94**, 578–596 (2009)
4. Vaillant, M., Glaunès, J.: Surface matching via currents. In: Christensen, G.E., Sonka, M. (eds.) IPMI 2005. LNCS, vol. 3565, pp. 381–392. Springer, Heidelberg (2005)
5. Mansi, T., Voigt, I., Leonardi, B., Pennec, X., Durrleman, S., Sermesant, M., Delingette, H., Taylor, A.M., Boudjemline, Y., Pongiglione, G., Ayache, N.: A statistical model for quantification and prediction of cardiac remodelling: application to tetralogy of fallot. IEEE Trans. Med. Imaging. **30**, 1605–1616 (2011)
6. Durrleman, S., Pennec, X., Trouvè, A., Ayache, N.: Statistical models of sets of curves and surfaces based on currents. Med. Image Anal. **13**, 793–808 (2009)
7. Ntsinjana, H.N., Biglino, G., Capelli, C., Tann, O., Giardini, A., Derrick, G., Schievano, S., Taylor, A.M.: Aortic arch shape is not associated with hypertensive response to exercise in patients with repaired congenital heart diseases. J. Cardiovasc. Magn. Reson. **15**, 101 (2013)
8. DuBois, D., DuBois, E.: The measurement of the surface area of man. Arch. Intern. Med. **15**(5), 869–881 (1915)
9. Antiga, L., Piccinelli, M., Botti, L., Ene-Iordache, B., Remuzzi, A., Steinman, D.A.: An image-based modeling framework for patient-specific computational hemodynamics. Med. Biol. Eng. Comput. **46**, 1097–1112 (2008)
10. Besl, P.J., McKay, N.D.: A method for registration of 3-D shapes. IEEE Trans. Pattern Anal. Mach. Intell. **14**, 239–256 (1992)
11. Tan, J.-L., Babu-Narayan, S.V., Henein, M.Y., Mullen, M., Li, W.: Doppler echocardiographic profile and indexes in the evaluation of aortic coarctation in patients before and after stenting. J. Am. Coll. Cardiol. **46**, 1045–1053 (2005)
12. Singh, N., Thomas Fletcher, P., Samuel Preston, J., King, R.D., Marron, J.S., Weiner, M.W., Joshi, S.: Quantifying anatomical shape variations in neurological disorders. Med. Image Anal. **18**, 616–633 (2014)

Towards Left Ventricular Scar Localisation Using Local Motion Descriptors

Devis Peressutti[1]([✉]), Wenjia Bai[2], Wenzhe Shi[2], Catalina Tobon-Gomez[1], Thomas Jackson[1], Manav Sohal[1], Aldo Rinaldi[1], Daniel Rueckert[2], and Andrew King[1]

[1] Division of Imaging Sciences and Biomedical Engineering, King's College London, London, UK
devis.1.peressutti@kcl.ac.uk
[2] Biomedical Image Analysis Group, Imperial College London, London, UK

Abstract. We propose a novel technique for the localisation of Left Ventricular (LV) scar based on local motion descriptors. Cardiac MR imaging is employed to construct a spatio-temporal motion atlas where the LV motion of different subjects can be directly compared. Local motion descriptors are derived from the motion atlas and dictionary learning is used for scar classification. Preliminary results on a cohort of 20 patients show a sensitivity and specificity of 80 % and 87 % in a binary classification setting.

1   Introduction

Accurate assessment of Left Ventricular (LV) scar location is paramount in many clinical applications, ranging from the evaluation of viable LV myocardium following myocardial infarction, to the planning of optimal lead placement in Cardiac Resynchronisation Therapy (CRT) or cardiac stem cells transplant [1,10].

Cardiac Magnetic Resonance (CMR) has become the imaging modality of choice for the characterisation of cardiac function and scar distribution due to its high spatial resolution, soft-tissue contrast and non-invasiveness. In particular, delayed-enhancement MR (DE-MR) imaging allows evaluation of the extent of scarred myocardium after injection of a contrast agent [10]. In DE-MR, scarred areas appear hyper-enhanced compared to healthy myocardium and scar transmurality is typically quantified by manually adjusting an intensity threshold. Standard clinical DE-MR protocols typically acquire 2D short-axis (SA) and long-axis (LA) images of the LV with slice thickness $\approx 10\,mm$, and therefore lack accurate through-plane scar information. Furthermore, DE-MR requires the use of a contrast agent, which is typically a gadolinium-based nephrotoxic drug.

Injured myocardium alters LV electrical activation and mechanical contraction, which causes differences in LV motion between ischaemic and non-ischaemic myocardium [7]. We present a framework for the prediction of LV scar location purely based on LV motion, without the need for a DE-MR scan or user interaction. We present preliminary results on a cohort of patients selected for CRT,

© Springer International Publishing Switzerland 2016
O. Camara et al. (Eds.): STACOM 2015, LNCS 9534, pp. 30–39, 2016.
DOI: 10.1007/978-3-319-28712-6_4

but the proposed framework has potential use in the assessment of LV scar distribution for other applications. To the authors' knowledge, very little work has been done on the use of 3D LV motion for automatic localisation of scar. Related work includes [8], in which the cardiac shape at different cardiac phases was used to characterise scarred myocardium, although it should be noted that their best results were achieved using the shape at only a single phase (end systole).

In the proposed method, LV motion is estimated using (T-MR) imaging, which provides 3D high-spatial resolution motion information. A spatio-temporal motion atlas is generated to remove biases towards LV geometry and cardiac cycle duration, allowing direct comparison of the LV motions of different patients. The novelty of our method lies in the use of local motion descriptors and dictionary learning to localise scar. Provided with the 3D LV motion descriptors of an unseen patient, the proposed framework is able to predict location of scarred myocardium.

2   Materials

A cohort of 20 patients[1] fulfilling conventional criteria for CRT (New York Heart Association functional classes II to IV, QRS duration $> 120\,ms$, and LV ejection fraction $\leq 35\,\%$) was considered. All patients underwent CMR imaging using a 1.5 T scanner (Achieva, Philips Healthcare, Best, Netherlands) with a 32-element cardiac coil. Details of the acquired CMR sequences are as follows:

cine MR: a multi-slice SA and three single-slice LA (2-chamber, 3-chamber and 4-chamber view) 2D cine Steady State Free Precession (SSFP) sequences were acquired (TR/TE $= 3.0/1.5\,ms$, flip angle $= 60°$). The SA and LA images have a typical slice thickness of $8\,mm$ and $10\,mm$, respectively and an in-plane resolution $\approx 1.4 \times 1.4\,mm^2$;

T-MR: tagged MR sequences in three orthogonal directions with reduced field-of-view enclosing the left ventricle were acquired (TR/TE $= 7.0/3.2\,ms$, flip angle $= 19$–$25°$, tag distance $= 7\,mm$). The data for each tagging direction consisted of multiple 2D slices covering the whole LV volume. The typical spatial resolution in the plane orthogonal to the tagging direction is $\approx 1.0 \times 1.0\,mm^2$;

DE-MR: delayed-enhancement MR images were acquired 15 to 20 min following the administration of 0.1 to $0.2\,mmol/kg$ gadopentate dimeglumine (Magnevist, Bayer Healthcare, Dublin, Ireland) using conventional inversion recovery sequences. A multi-slice SA and three single-slice LA 2D images were acquired (TR/TE $= 5.6/2.0\,ms$, flip angle $= 25°$). The same field-of-view and orientation as the cine MR sequences was used. Slice thickness of both SA and LA images is $10\,mm$ with an in-plane resolution $\approx 1.4 \times 1.4\,mm^2$.

All images were acquired during sequential breath-holds of approximately $15\,s$ and were ECG-gated. Given their high in-plane spatial resolution, the cine

---

[1] Data were acquired from different projects and cannot be made publicly available due to lack of ethical approval or patient consent on data sharing.

MR images at end-diastole (ED) were employed to estimate LV geometry (see Sect. 3.1). The other cine MR images were not used in this work. An average high resolution $3D + t$ T-MR sequence was derived from the three T-MR acquisitions with orthogonal tagging directions and was used to estimate the LV deformation (see Sect. 3.1). Finally, the DE-MR images were used to estimate the location of LV scar. These scar maps were used in the training and validation of the classifier (see Sect. 3.2).

3   Methods

The main novelty of the proposed method lies in the application of dictionary learning to 3D LV motion descriptors for classification of scarred myocardium. An illustration of the proposed framework is shown in Fig. 1. To allow motion comparison from different patients, a spatio-temporal motion atlas of the LV was generated similarly to [4]. The use of a spatio-temporal motion atlas allowed us to remove differences in LV anatomy and cardiac cycle duration from the comparison of LV motion.

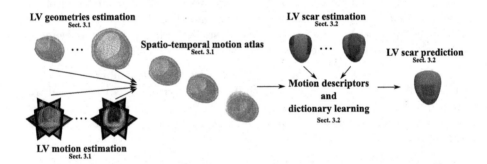

Fig. 1. Overview of the proposed framework.

3.1   Spatio-Temporal Motion Atlas

The formation of the LV spatio-temporal motion atlas comprises estimation of LV geometry and motion, spatial normalisation of LV geometries and motion reorientation from each subject-specific to the common atlas coordinate system.

Prior to the LV geometry and motion estimation, the SA and LA cine MR sequences were spatially aligned to the T-MR coordinate system, as in [11].

LV Geometry Estimation. For each patient, the end-diastolic (ED) cardiac phase was chosen as the temporal reference. The LV myocardium, excluding papillary muscles, was manually segmented from the ED frames of the multi-slice SA and three LA cine MR images. The four binary masks were fused together into an isotropic $2\,mm^3$ binary image and the result was further refined manually to obtain a smooth LV segmentation. To determine point correspondences amongst all LV geometries, an open-source statistical shape model (SSM) of the LV was employed [6]. The SSM represents the anatomical variance of a population of 134 patients and consists of the epi- and endo-cardial surfaces. After an initial landmark-based rigid alignment, the modes of variation of the SSM were optimised to maximise the overlap between the LV segmentation and the volume of the SSM. Non-rigid registration followed the mode optimisation to refine local alignment. An example of a resulting LV surface is shown in Fig. 2(a), (b), (c), (d), (e), (f) and (g).

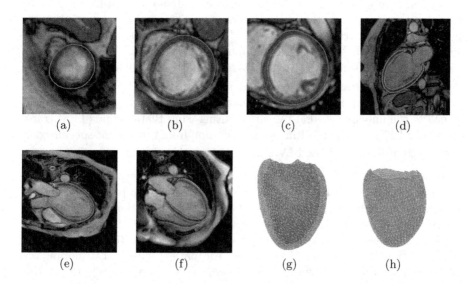

(a)   (b)   (c)   (d)

(e)   (f)   (g)   (h)

Fig. 2. Example of estimated LV anatomical surface at end-diastole. The estimated LV mesh is overlaid onto a (a) apical, (b) mid and (c) basal cine SA slice and (d) 2-chamber, (e) 3-chamber, and (f) 4-chamber cine LA slices. Figure (g) shows the resulting SSM epi- and endo-cardial meshes, while (h) shows the resampled medial LV mesh.

To facilitate the computation of motion descriptors, a medial surface mesh with regularly sampled vertices ($\approx$1500) was generated from the personalised SSM epi- and endo-cardial surfaces. An example of a resampled medial surface is shown in Fig. 2(h). The same resampling strategy was employed for all patients to maintain point correspondence.

LV Motion Estimation. As mentioned in Sect. 2, an average high resolution $3D+t$ T-MR sequence was derived from the $3D+t$ T-MR sequences with orthogonal tagging planes. For each patient, the trigger time t_T specified in the DICOM meta-tag of the T-MR volumes was normalised with respect to the patient's average cardiac cycle, such that $t_T \in [0, 1)$, with 0 being ED. A $3D + t$ free-form-deformation algorithm with sparse spatial and temporal constraints [12] was employed to estimate LV motion with respect to the ED cardiac phase.

This algorithm estimates a smooth and continuous $3D + t$ transformation for any $t \in [0, 1)$. This way, temporal normalisation was achieved for each patient, regardless of the number of acquired T-MR volumes and cycle length.

Spatial Normalisation. Spatial normalisation aims to remove bias towards patient-specific LV geometries from the motion analysis. LV surfaces at ED (see Fig. 2(h)) were derived from N patients using the steps outlined above. An initial Procrustes alignment based on the point correspondences was performed on the N medial LV surfaces, obtaining a set of affine transformations $\{\phi_{aff}^n\}, n = 1, \ldots, N$ with respect to a randomly chosen reference. An average surface was computed from the aligned surfaces and an unbiased LV medial surface was computed by transforming the average surface by the inverse of the average affine transformation $\tilde{\phi}_{aff} = \frac{1}{n} \sum_n \phi_{aff}^n$. This way, bias towards the initial reference is removed. An example of an unbiased LV surface is shown in Fig. 3(b). The original transformations $\{\phi_{aff}^n\}$ were similarly normalised to enforce an average similarity transformation equal to identity $\hat{\phi}_{aff}^n = \phi_{aff}^n \circ (\tilde{\phi}_{aff})^{-1}$. To capture the local differences in LV geometry, all surfaces were consequently aligned to the unbiased medial LV surface using Thin Plate Spline (TPS) transformations $\{\phi_{TPS}^n\}$. The resulting transformation from the patient-specific coordinate system to the unbiased LV surface is given by $\phi^n = \phi_{TPS}^n \circ \hat{\phi}_{aff}^n$ [4].

Motion Reorientation. To compare cardiac phases amongst all patients, the reference ED medial surface was warped to $T = 24$ cardiac phases equally distributed in $[0, 0.8]$ by using the estimated $3D + t$ transformation for each patient. Only the first 80 % of the cardiac cycle was considered since it is the typical coverage of T-MR sequences, and the estimated motion for $t \in (0.8, 1]$ is therefore due to motion interpolation. As a result, the patient-specific LV motion was fully represented by the T shapes. We denote with $\mathbf{v}_{p,t}^n = \mathbf{u}_{p,t}^n - \mathbf{u}_{p,0}^n$ the motion at location $\mathbf{u}$ of vertex $p \in 1, .., P$ at the cardiac phase $t \in 1, .., T$ with respect to the ED phase for patient $n \in 1, .., N$. The aim of motion reorientation is to transport $\mathbf{v}_{p,t}^n, \forall n, t, p$ from each patient specific coordinate system to the coordinate system of the unbiased average surface. Under a small displacement assumption [3,9], this is achieved by computing $\mathbf{v}_{n,p,t}^{atlas} = J^{-1}(\phi^n(\mathbf{u}_p)) \cdot \mathbf{v}_{p,t}^n$, where $J(\phi^n)$ denotes the Jacobian of the transformation ϕ^n [3,4,9]. After reorientation, LV motion from different patients can be directly compared at each vertex p of the unbiased LV medial surface and cardiac phase t.

3.2 Local Motion Descriptors

As a result of the previous steps, the LV motions $\mathbf{v}_{n,p,t}^{atlas}, \forall n, p, t$ are represented in a common coordinate system. For a better description of the LV motion, the atlas was segmented into the standard 16 AHA segments [2] (see Fig. 3(a) and (b)) and the LV motions $\mathbf{v}_{n,p,t}^{atlas}$ were decomposed into longitudinal, radial and circumferential cylindrical coordinates ($\mathbf{v}_{n,p,t}^{atlas} = [l_{n,p,t}, r_{n,p,t}, c_{n,p,t}]^T$) with respect to the long axis of the LV ED medial surface.

For each patient, the LV scar distribution was estimated from the SA and LA DE-MR images by using cmr^{42} (Circle Cardiovascular Imaging Inc.). The software requires the observer to delineate the endo- and epi-cardial LV contours and to set an intensity threshold to best separate scarred from healthy myocardium. In this work, a single clinical expert derived the scar maps to eliminate inter-observer variability. Figure 3(c) shows an example of a resulting scar map, where the scar transmurality is specified for each AHA segment, while Fig. 3(d) shows the scar distribution mapped onto the unbiased LV atlas.

The aim of this work is to characterise scar as a function of the LV spatio-temporal motion information. To this end, as described in Guha *et al.* [5], local motion pattern (LMP) descriptors were computed from the spatio-temporal motion atlas to characterise the scar, and dictionary learning was subsequently employed on the LMP descriptors for classification. Finally, in order to robustly cope with outliers, a Random Sample Reconstruction [5] was employed to localise the scar of an unseen patient.

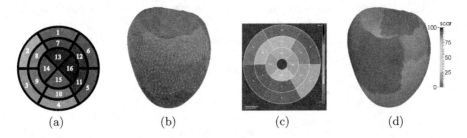

(a)   (b)   (c)   (d)

Fig. 3. The standard AHA bull's eye plot (a) and the segmented unbiased LV medial mesh at ED (b). An example of scar distribution provided by the software cmr^{42} and mapped onto the atlas is shown in (c)–(d)

Local Motion Pattern Descriptors. A LMP descriptor represents the local variations of the LV in the spatio-temporal dimensions [5]. After normalisation of the LV motions $\mathbf{v}_{n,p,t}^{atlas}$ with respect to the temporal norm $\|\mathbf{v}_{n,p}^{atlas}\|$, a neighbourhood B_p for each vertex p was considered. LMP descriptors were computed as the concatenation of the first 4 central temporal moments (mean, variance, skewness and kurtosis) for the circumferential, radial and longitudinal components for each point $p_i \in B_p$ at different temporal intervals (see Fig. 4). The three components were treated separately, as evidence has shown the different impact of the components on scar characterisation [7]. This results in a matrix $\mathbf{X} \in \mathbb{R}^{(M) \times (NP)}$, where M is proportional to the number of temporal intervals and the size of the neighbourhood (see Fig. 4). Given the high dimensionality of the LMP descriptors, Random Projections were used to reduce the complexity of the classification task, resulting in a matrix $\mathbf{\Psi} \in \mathbb{R}^{(D) \times (NP)}, D \ll M$, which contains projections of $\mathbf{X}$ onto a random D-dimensional subspace [5].

Concatenated Dictionary Learning. Dictionary learning (DL) techniques can learn an overcomplete set of basis functions (i.e. dictionary) to represent a signal with a high level of sparsity. DL has been employed successfully in many image processing tasks, including denoising, inpainting and classification.

In our context, the scar transmurality was divided into K evenly distributed classes within the $0-100\%$ scar transmurality range and the sparsity properties of DL were exploited for classification. In particular, a concatenated DL technique was employed under the hypothesis that LMP descriptors of scar class k are better represented by the corresponding dictionary rather than a dictionary of a different class. Therefore, class-specific dictionaries were trained by solving

$$\langle \boldsymbol{\Phi}_k, \mathbf{S}_k \rangle = \underset{\boldsymbol{\Phi}_k, \mathbf{S}_k}{argmin} \|\boldsymbol{\Psi}_k - \boldsymbol{\Phi}_k \mathbf{S}_k\|_2^2 + \alpha \|\mathbf{S}_k\|_1, \qquad (1)$$

where $\boldsymbol{\Psi}_k \in \mathbb{R}^{(D) \times (NP)_k}$, $\boldsymbol{\Phi}_k \in \mathbb{R}^{(D) \times (A)}$ and $\mathbf{S}_k \in \mathbb{R}^{(A) \times (NP)_k}$ respectively are the descriptor matrix, the dictionary and the sparse code for the scar class k, while A is the number of basis functions (i.e. atoms) and $(NP)_k$ is the number of points belonging to the scar class k. We denote by $\langle .. \rangle$ the variables being optimised. The $scikit - learn$ python package was used for the code implementation and a least angle regression method was used to solve the lasso problem. After training, the K dictionaries were concatenated into a single dictionary $\boldsymbol{\Phi}_C = [\boldsymbol{\Phi}_1|...|\boldsymbol{\Phi}_K]$ and, provided with a set of unseen descriptors $\boldsymbol{\Psi}_{un}$, the sparse code $\mathbf{S}_{un}$ was computed using the Orthogonal Matching Pursuit (OMP) greedy algorithm for the optimisation of

$$\langle \mathbf{S}_{un} \rangle = \underset{\mathbf{S}_{un}}{argmin} \|\boldsymbol{\Psi}_{un} - \boldsymbol{\Phi}_C \mathbf{S}_{un}\|_2^2, \quad s.t. \quad \|\mathbf{s}_{un}\|_0 \le \beta. \qquad (2)$$

The sparse code $\mathbf{S}_{un}$ is the concatenation of $[\mathbf{S}_{\boldsymbol{\Phi}_1}|...|\mathbf{S}_{\boldsymbol{\Phi}_K}]$ where $\mathbf{S}_{\boldsymbol{\Phi}_k}$ is the sparse code corresponding to $\boldsymbol{\Phi}_k$. The estimated scar class is

$$k_e = \underset{i \in 1,..,K}{argmax} \|\mathbf{S}_{\boldsymbol{\Phi}_i}\|_0, \qquad (3)$$

where $\|\mathbf{S}_{\boldsymbol{\Phi}_i}\|_0$ counts the non-zero entries of $\mathbf{S}_{\boldsymbol{\Phi}_i}$ [5].

Since the scar size can vary within a given AHA segment, the classification was performed using a Random Sample Reconstruction (RSR) [5], where the class k_e is assigned to the AHA segment if a randomly chosen subset of descriptors also belongs to the same class. RSR provides robustness to the classification, allowing classification of whole AHA segments based on a smaller set of descriptive points, as is the case for localised scarred myocardium (see [5] for details).

4   Experiments and Results

Given the low number of datasets containing scar in the apical and basal segments, the AHA segments corresponding to the LV mid cavity only (i.e. segments 7 to 12) were analysed. On average, each segment contained ≈ 100 points. For

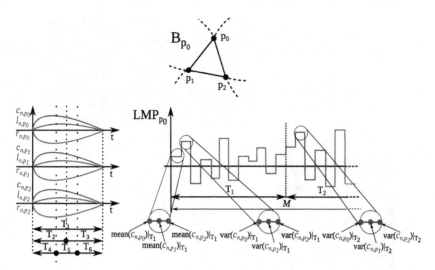

Fig. 4. Toy example of LMP descriptor computation for a neighbourhood composed of 3 points ($B_{p_0} = 3$). The descriptor is derived by concatenating the first four central moments of the circumferential (blue), radial (green) and longitudinal (red) components for each $p_i \in B_p, i = 1, 2, 3$ computed over 6 temporal intervals $T_j, j = 1, ..6$ (Color figure online).

simplicity, a binary classification (i.e. K=2, 0 - no scar, 1 - scar) was considered. The distribution of the binary ground-truth scar over all patients within the considered segments is shown in Fig. 5(a).

A leave-one-out cross validation was employed. Given the high number of free parameters for our technique, the best set was determined empirically, since an exhaustive search proved to be cumbersome. The set of parameters used was: $B_p = 8, j = 6$ temporal intervals (see Fig. 4), $D = 256$, sparsity coefficient $\alpha = .5$, maximum number of iterations $= 200$, number of atoms $A = 512$, number of non-zero coefficients in OMP $\beta = 2$. For the RSR, random set size ≈ 5 descriptors, probability of selecting an error-free set of points $P = .9$ (see [5]).

Results of the binary classification are reported in Fig. 5 considering each segment as an independent observation. Values of sensitivity, specificity, positive predictive value (PPV) and negative predictive value (NPV) achieved were 80 %, 87 %, 36 % and 98 %, respectively.

5 Discussion

In this paper, a novel framework for LV scar location using local motion descriptors has been proposed. Results on a cohort of 20 patients enrolled for CRT treatment were presented, with a sensitivity and specificity of 80 % and 87 % in a binary scar classification setting. Although the investigation presented in this paper is preliminary, to the authors' knowledge this is the first work to demonstrate that scar can be localised using motion information alone. Therefore, this

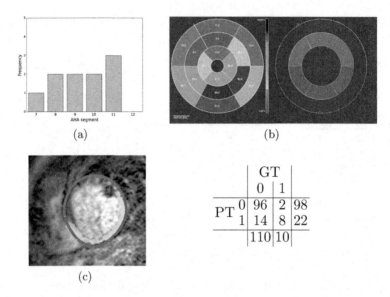

(a) (b)

(c)

	GT		
	0	1	
PT 0	96	2	98
PT 1	14	8	22
	110	10	

Fig. 5. (a) Scar distribution over AHA segments 7–12 (mid LV cavity). (b) Bull's eye plot of a GT map and predicted scar (0 - red, 1 - blue), mid-cavity segments only. (c) the corresponding predicted scar mapped onto the medial surface is overlaid onto the SA DE-MR image (the LV scar in yellow). (Bottom right) Joint frequency table of AHA segment classification (GT - ground-truth, PT - proposed technique) (Color figure online).

represents an important proof-of-principle that such a technique may one day aid or even replace DE-MR in LV scar localisation and quantification.

There are a number of areas for future investigation before this possibility might become reality. One is the use of a larger number of scar classes (i.e. not a binary classification), or even a regression-based approach in which scar transmurality is directly predicted from the LMP descriptors. Further work is also required to refine the localisation of the ground truth scar, in which transmurality is currently assigned for all points within a segment. Moreover, inter- and intra- observer variability in the determination of scar transmurality needs to be investigated. Finally, investigations using larger numbers of scar-affected datasets is required.

Acknowledgements. This work was funded by EPSRC Grants EP/K030310/1 and EP/K030523/1. We acknowledge financial support from the Department of Health via the NIHR comprehensive Biomedical Research Centre award to Guy's & St Thomas' NHS Foundation Trust with KCL and King's College Hospital NHS Foundation Trust.

References

1. Bilchick, K.C., Kuruvilla, S., Hamirani, Y.S., Ramachandran, R., Clarke, S.A., Parker, K.M., Stukenborg, G.J., Mason, P., Ferguson, J.D., Moorman, J.R., Malhotra, R., Mangrum, J.M., Darby, A.E., DiMarco, J., Holmes, J.W., Salerno, M., Kramer, C.M., Epstein, F.H.: Impact of mechanical activation, scar, and electrical timing on cardiac resynchronization therapy response and clinical outcomes. J. Am. Coll. Cardiol. **63**(16), 1657–1666 (2014)
2. Cerqueira, M.D., Weissman, N.J., Dilsizian, V., Jacobs, A.K., Kaul, S., Laskey, W.K., Pennell, D.J., Rumberger, J.A., Ryan, T., Verani, M.S.: Standardized myocardial segmentation and nomenclature for tomographic imaging of the heart. Circulation **105**(4), 539–542 (2002)
3. Chandrashekara, R., Rao, A., Sanchez-Ortiz, G.I., Mohiaddin, R.H., Rueckert, D.: Construction of a statistical model for cardiac motion analysis using nonrigid image registration. In: Taylor, C.J., Noble, J.A. (eds.) IPMI 2003. LNCS, vol. 2732, pp. 599–610. Springer, Heidelberg (2003)
4. De Craene, M., Duchateau, N., Tobon-Gomez, C., Ghafaryasl, B., Piella, G., Rhode, K.S., Frange, A.: SPM to the heart: Mapping of 4D continuous velocities for motion abnormality quantification. In: Proc. of IEEE ISBI, pp. 454–457 (2012)
5. Guha, T., Ward, R.: Learning sparse representations for human action recognition. IEEE Trans. Pattern Anal. Mach. Intell. **34**(8), 1576–1588 (2012)
6. Hoogendoorn, C., Duchateau, N., Sanchez-Quintana, D., Whitmarsh, T., Sukno, F., De Craene, M., Lekadir, K., Frangi, A.: A high-resolution atlas and statistical model of the human heart from multislice CT. IEEE Trans. Med. Imaging **32**(1), 28–44 (2013)
7. Maret, E., Todt, T., Brudin, L., Nylander, E., Swahn, E., Ohlsson, J., Engvall, J.: Functional measurements based on feature tracking of cine magnetic resonance images identify left ventricular segments with myocardial scar. Cardiovasc. Ultrasound **7**(1), 53 (2009)
8. Medrano-Gracia, P., Suinesiaputra, A., Cowan, B., Bluemke, D., Frangi, A., Lee, D., Lima, J., Young, A.: An atlas for cardiac MRI regional wall motion and infarct scoring. In: Camara, O., Mansi, T., Pop, M., Rhode, K., Sermesant, M., Young, A. (eds.) STACOM 2012. LNCS, vol. 7746, pp. 188–197. Springer, Heidelberg (2013)
9. Rao, A., Chandrashekara, R., Sanchez-Ortiz, G., Mohiaddin, R., Aljabar, P., Hajnal, J., Puri, B.K., Rueckert, D.: Spatial transformation of motion and deformation fields using nonrigid registration. IEEE Trans. Med. Imaging **23**(9), 1065–1076 (2004)
10. Shan, K., Constantine, G., Sivananthan, M., Flamm, S.D.: Role of cardiac magnetic resonance imaging in the assessment of myocardial viability. Circulation **109**(11), 1328–1334 (2004)
11. Shi, W., Zhuang, X., Wang, H., Duckett, S., Luong, D., Tobon-Gomez, C., Tung, K., Edwards, P., Rhode, K., Razavi, R., Ourselin, S., Rueckert, D.: A comprehensive cardiac motion estimation framework using both untagged and 3-D tagged MR images based on nonrigid registration. IEEE Trans. Med. Imaging **31**(6), 1263–1275 (2012)
12. Shi, W., Jantsch, M., Aljabar, P., Pizarro, L., Bai, W., Wang, H., O'Regan, D., Zhuang, X., Rueckert, D.: Temporal sparse free-form deformations. Med. Image Anal. **17**(7), 779–789 (2013)

Traversed Graph Representation for Sparse Encoding of Macro-Reentrant Tachycardia

Mihaela Constantinescu[1]($\boxtimes$), Su-Lin Lee[1], Sabine Ernst[2],
and Guang-Zhong Yang[1]

[1] The Hamlyn Centre for Robotic Surgery, Imperial College London, London, UK
`mihaela.constantinescu12@imperial.ac.uk`
[2] The Royal Brompton and Harefield Hospital, London, UK

Abstract. Macro-reentrant atrial and ventricular tachycardias originate from additional circuits in which the activation of the cardiac chambers follows a high-frequency rotating pattern. The macro-reentrant circuit can be interrupted by targeted radiofrequency energy delivery with a linear lesion transecting the pathway. The choice of the optimal ablation site is determined by the operator's experience, thus limiting the procedure success, increasing its duration and also unnecessarily extending the ablated tissue area in the case of incorrect ablation target estimation. In this paper, an algorithm for automatic intraoperative detection of the tachycardia reentry path is proposed by modelling the propagation as a graph traverse problem. Moreover, the optimal ablation point where the path should be transected is computed. Finally, the proposed method is applied to sparse electroanatomical data to demonstrate its use when undersampled mapping occurs. Thirteen electroanatomical maps of right ventricle and right and left atrium tachycardias from patients treated for congenital heart disease were analysed retrospectively in this study, with prediction accuracy tested against the recorded ablation sites and arrhythmia termination points.

1 Introduction

In recent years, catheter ablation of cardiac arrhythmias has moved from ablation of 'simple' substrates like accessory pathways to more complex arrhythmias such as atrial or ventricular tachycardia or fibrillation. Even patients with complex congenital heart disease (CHD) that may present with a very unusual cardiac anatomy can now be candidates for catheter ablation procedures. Merging pre-procedural 3D image data with the 3D electroanatomy has provided a very valuable tool to improve ablation outcomes even during longterm follow-up.

The state-of-the-art in intraoperative guidance for mapping and ablating tachycardias in CHD includes CARTO (Biosense Webster, Bar Diamond, CA, US). After vascular access into the cardiac chamber, the mapping catheter is moved in contact with the endocardial wall in order to generate the spatial information, i.e. the fast anatomical map (FAM), and also acquire sparse electrical data at specifically selected points on the FAM. The electrical parameters

© Springer International Publishing Switzerland 2016
O. Camara et al. (Eds.): STACOM 2015, LNCS 9534, pp. 40–50, 2016.
DOI: 10.1007/978-3-319-28712-6_5

include unipolar and bipolar voltage and local activation times (LAT). With each point acquisition, CARTO interpolates the electrical parameters across the FAM using a preset distance threshold. From the LAT map, CARTO is able to simulate the activation wave based on a sequential plot of activation time geodesics. Apart from CARTO, a second widely used electroanatomical mapping system is EnSite NavX (St. Jude Medical, St. Paul, MN, US), which outputs the same activation time and voltage maps as CARTO, but employs a different technology. Despite the advances in these two systems, establishing the path of fastest conduction, i.e. the main ectopic propagation circuit, and correlating it with the location of fibrotic tissue shown on the bipolar voltage map are still operator-dependent skills.

Intra-operatively, the electrophysiologists guide themselves in locating the circuit by circuit entrainment mapping. They measure the post pacing interval at the reset of the tachycardia to see if the circuit was entered successfully. Naturally, with increasing numbers of mapping and pacing points, the activation and voltage amplitude maps become more accurate. However, there is a trade-off between mapping time and resolution. Moreover, if the ablation site is, by error or misinterpretation of the mapping data, far from the conduction path, repeated energy delivery will be required, causing more tissue damage than necessary. Successful ablation is declared if the mapped tachycardia is terminated during energy delivery and no longer inducible.

In order to understand the underlying mechanisms of macro-reentrant tachycardias, different electrophysiological models have been proposed for simulation. These models are meant to replace to some extent the more expensive electroanatomical mapping systems. They use general electrical wave propagation principles applied to the cardiac tissue and anatomy and personalised with electromechanical parameters from preoperative imaging. Although the well-established CARTO and EnSite technologies are preferred in clinical practice, the electroanatomical models can also provide the cardiologists with activation time maps and potentially voltage information. Among the least computationally expensive frameworks are the eikonal model for conduction parameter estimation at macro-scale [1,2], but also simplified biophysical ionic channel models [3] or mono-domain models such as Lattice-Boltzmann [4]. Fast Marching, an adaptation of the graph traverse Dijkstra algorithm, is typically used to solve the differential equations in these models. The solution of these equations can be mapped on 3D anatomy in order to mimic the information output of electroanatomical mapping systems. Alternatives to these classical biophysical approaches are the models of propagation in cellular automata [5] and the estimation of pathways as a minimal cost graph traverse formulation [6], the latter having been used for qualitative identification of the normal conduction along the Purkinje fibres.

This paper proposes a novel approach for the detection of tachycardia propagation path based on graph traverse theory by using the mapping data directly and without the need for simulation or electroanatomical model fitting. Furthermore, the point in the circuit of the highest termination probability was computed. The algorithms were tested for repeatability in sparse mapping conditions when fewer points are acquired. The proposed method was validated with data from 13 patients with previous CHD surgery and suffering from atrial or ventricular reentrant tachycardias.

2 Methods

2.1 Data Acquisition

CARTO 3 studies of macro-reentrant right ventricular and left and right atrial tachycardia were collected – 4 right ventricles, 6 right atria, 2 left atria, 1 total cavopulmonary connection (TCPC). Each study contained a 3D endocardial surface of the cardiac chamber, with a corresponding set of LATs, bipolar voltages, and unipolar voltages for each surface vertex. The anatomical meshes were smoothed with Poisson reconstruction, threshold set as the default 6, in Mesh-Lab [7]. The electrical data at the new vertices were interpolated linearly from the values on the original meshes. The latest and earliest activation times with respect to the end-diastolic ECG peak (R peak) were extracted. The input data required by the proposed method is independent of the CARTO system, as long as the electroanatomical information can be recovered with another technology, e.g. EnSite, or modelled using any cardiac activation principles.

2.2 Macro-Reentrant Circuit Reconstruction

For macro-reentrant circuit reconstruction, the shortest geodesic path between the earliest and the latest activation vertices was computed. The mesh edges were used as graph edges and the vertices as nodes. The edges were weighted with the propagation speed between the vertices that they connected, multiplied by the means of the bipolar and unipolar voltage amplitudes at the two vertices (Eq. 1).

$$
w_{i,j} = \frac{d_{i,j}}{|\mathrm{LAT}_i - \mathrm{LAT}_j|} \cdot \frac{V_{\mathrm{uni},i} + V_{\mathrm{uni},j}}{2} \cdot \frac{V_{\mathrm{bi},i} + V_{\mathrm{bi},j}}{2} \tag{1}
$$

The variable $w_{i,j}$ is the weight of the edge connecting vertex i to vertex j, each with activation times LAT_i and LAT_j, unipolar voltage amplitudes $V_{\mathrm{uni},i}$ and $V_{\mathrm{uni},j}$, and bipolar voltage amplitudes $V_{\mathrm{bi},i}$ and $V_{\mathrm{bi},j}$. The propagation speed between the neighbouring vertices i and j was computed from the Euclidean distance $d_{i,j}$. The product of mean voltage amplitudes modelled the energy of the wave traversing that part of the tissue, dependent on the tissue conductivity. This modulated the path to avoid crossing areas of surgical scars, which have low conductivity. Finally, Dijkstra's algorithm was applied [8].

Due to the limitations of the interpolation algorithm in CARTO, the earliest and latest activation points may not directly coincide, leaving a strip of artificially interpolated LATs (Fig. 1). Also in some cases, the incomplete geometry of the endocardial chamber caused the activation circuit to be represented only partially. The remaining gap was closed with a new application of the Dijkstra algorithm on the complementary path, which was forced to pass through the vertex opposite to the centre of the path found in the first Dijkstra run.

2.3   Tachycardia Termination Point Detection

The electrical features of typical tachycardia points were learned and tested in a leave-one-out fashion. For each of the 13 studies, the triplets of LAT, bipolar voltages, and unipolar voltages of the points along the path were normalised and concatenated. The LATs were a measure of position of the termination points along the parameterised path running from earliest to latest activation; the voltages were a measure of tissue fibrosis. Each study was left out in turn from the full set of 13. The points on the remaining 12 paths were fed as a training set into an adapted version of a random subsampling boosting classifier (RUSBoost, presented in [9] and adapted as in Algorithm 1).

The labels of the training set were exported from CARTO and projected onto the paths, in order to distinguish between the features of the two classes, ablation points and regular points. The learner predicted the labels of the path points on the test case. RUSBoost was deemed the most adequate classification method given the imbalanced number of termination points compared to the other points on the path.

Data:
- $(y_{\text{train},i}, \text{LAT}_{\text{train},i}, \text{bi}_{\text{train},i}, \text{uni}_{\text{train},i})$, $i = \overline{1, n_{\text{train}}}$ and $y_{\text{train},i} \in \{0, 1\}$, where 0 denotes regular path point and 1 termination point, as marked in CARTO
- number of termination points is significantly lower than the number of regular path points, i.e. $n_1 \ll n_0$
- $(\text{LAT}_{\text{test},i}, \text{bi}_{\text{test},i}, \text{uni}_{\text{test},i})$, $i = \overline{1, n_{\text{test}}}$
- weak learner, which does not necessarily yield a good initial classification.

Initialization: $w_{1,i} = \frac{1}{n_{\text{train}}}, i = \overline{1, n_{\text{train}}}$, where $w_{k,i}$ is the weight of sample i in iteration k;
while *preset number of iterations not reached* **do**

    1. subsample from the full set using the weights $w_{k,i}$, $i = \overline{1, n_{\text{train}}}$;
    2. feed the subset and the weights to the learner;
    3. learner estimates the labels of the training data;
    4. update the weights with the classification error;

end
Result: $y_{\text{test},i} = 0$ or $y_{\text{test},i} = 1$, $p(y_{\text{test},i} = 1)$, and $p(y_{\text{test},i} \neq 1)$, where $i = \overline{1, n_{\text{test}}}$

Algorithm 1. RUSBoost classification algorithm for detection of most probable point of tachycardia termination

2.4   Subsampling of Electroanatomical Maps

Electrical Data Interpolation. In order to test how the circuit reconstruction and the termination point detection perform on sparse electroanatomical data, subsampling of the original maps was performed. The electrical values of every vertex in the sparse maps were obtained through a two-step interpolation and threshold filling algorithm, tuned to mimic the online interpolation of CARTO when new electroanatomical data is acquired.

In the first step, for every vertex, only the mapping points within a 12 mm radius were taken into consideration. The value at that vertex was either that of the mapping points, if it coincided, or the mean of the values of all mapping points within 12 mm, weighted inversely with the distance from the vertex. In the second step, the vertices which did not have any mapping points to meet the proximity threshold were given the value of their closest vertex with an assigned value from the interpolation step. The value of 12 mm was set by trial and error to best match the CARTO ground truth. A qualitative comparison can be made between the figures in Table 2 and the original mesh in Fig. 1.

Iterative Cluster Subsampling. The original mapping points were clustered around 5 centroids computed with the k-means method and approximated by the closest mapping point in the cluster according to the Cartesian distance. The 5 centroids were ordered using a greedy search with respect to their marginal information, which is explained in the next paragraphs.

Given the full set of mapping points P_0, from which the ground-truth electroanatomical map was built, and a subset $P \subset P_0$, the map reconstruction accuracy when using subset P for interpolation can be computed as the inverse of the error

$$\varepsilon_{P \sim P_0} = \frac{1}{3} \sum_{i \in \{LAT, uni, bi\}} \frac{1}{j} \sum_{j=1}^{n_V} \frac{|f_{i,j,P} - f_{i,j,P_0}|}{\max_{i,j} f_{i,j,P_0} - \min_{i,j} f_{i,j,P_0}}. \qquad (2)$$

The anatomy is in both cases a 3D surface of n_V vertices. The value $f_{i,j}, i \in \{LAT, uni, bi\}$, is either the LAT, unipolar voltage (uni), or bipolar (bi) voltage at vertex j. For each vertex, the difference in electroanatomical values was scaled with reference to the P_0 map. The marginal information of a mapping point can be defined as the difference in map accuracy between two maps constructed with and without that particular point. The adapted greedy search for ordering the centroids according to their marginal information is presented in Algorithm 2.

The path reconstruction and termination point detection were run in 5 iterations, where in each iteration a new cluster of points was added to interpolate the colour maps.

3   Results

3.1   Macro-Reentrant Circuit Reconstruction

For each of the 13 cases, the graph was built with the FAM vertices and edges. The forward circuit was computed using Matlab's implementation of the Dijkstra algorithm with weights as in Eq. 1. Figure 1 shows qualitative results on a right ventricle and on left and right atria. The CARTO ablation, circuit entrainment, and termination points are displayed as reference points of the ground-truth propagation path detected intraoperatively. The dense bipolar voltage maps were

Data:

- P_0 full set of mapping points;
- f_{i,j,P_0}, $i \in \{\text{LAT}, \text{uni}, \text{bi}\}$, $j = \overline{1, n_V}$, electrical features of all vertices for the map computed with the points in P_0
- vertex indices of the 5 centroids

Initialization: $c_1 = \arg\min_k \varepsilon_{(P_0 - \{k\}) \sim P_0}$, $k = \overline{1,5}$;
while $i <=$ *number of clusters - 1* **do**

    1. interpolate for $f_{i,j,\{c_{\overline{1,i}}\}}$ and $f_{i,j,(\{c_{\overline{1,i}}\} \cup \{k\})}$, where $k = \overline{1,5} - \{c_{\overline{1,i}}\}$;

    2. $c_{i+1} = \arg\max_k |\varepsilon_{\{c_{\overline{1,i}}\} \sim P_0} - \varepsilon_{(\{c_{\overline{1,i}}\} \cup \{k\}) \sim P_0}|$;

    3. $i = i + 1$;

end
Result: c, decreasing order of centroid marginal information

Algorithm 2. Ordering of the cluster centroids according to their marginal information added to the electroanatomical map

thresholded at 0.5 mV, a value commonly used in the EP literature for ventricular scar segmentation in electroanatomic data. The third row of results, displayed on top of the scar maps, shows that the calculation of propagation paths avoids the crossing of scars, according to the edge weights in Eq. 1.

Several qualitative observations can be made from the results shown in Fig. 1. Firstly, there was a good correlation between the LAT geodesics and the computed path perpendicular to them. Secondly, the paths were modulated by the presence of surgical scar, encoded by the bipolar voltage amplitude at each vertex. The perpendicularity of the paths to the LAT geodesics is ensured by the core principle of shortest path in the Dijkstra algorithm.

Table 1 shows a quantitative analysis of both tachycardia circuit detection and termination point learning. Assuming that all critical points labelled intra-operatively and imported from CARTO, i.e. circuit entrainment, ablation, and final tachycardia termination points, lie on the true wave propagation path, an accuracy measure was defined as the distance between this ground-truth and the computed path, namely the mean distance to CARTO points. The average of 16.36 mm was comparable to the range of tip instability of the ablation catheter (12 mm), as recorded by the electromagnetic sensors in the CARTO framework.

3.2 Tachycardia Termination Point Detection

Several measures were defined to assess the method's performance in this step: the accuracy, sensitivity, and specificity, all of which quantified the ability to distinguish a regular path point from an critical point on the path. A critical point is either an ablation, a termination, or a circuit entrainment point as labelled and exported from CARTO. A critical path point is the projection of a critical point onto the tachycardia path reconstructed in the first step of the method.

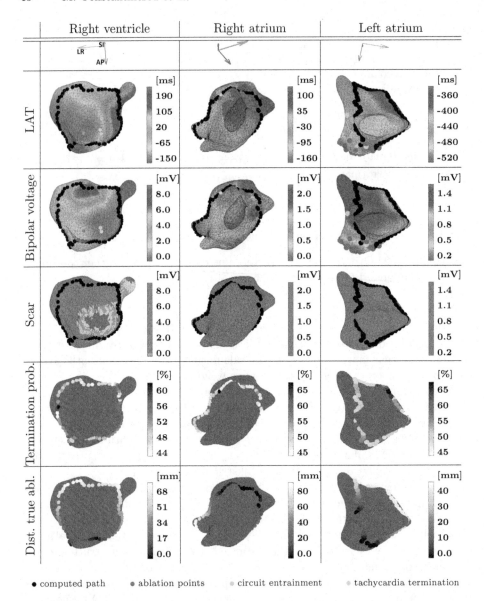

● computed path   ● ablation points   ● circuit entrainment   ● tachycardia termination

Fig. 1. Tachycardia propagation path for average right and left atria and for an average right ventricle. The panels show from top to bottom the LAT, bipolar voltage, and scar maps, the probability of tachycardia termination at each point along the path, and the distance of the computed termination points from the closest ground-truth ablation. AP – antero-posterior axis, LR – left-right axis, SI – supero-inferior axis.

Apart from the relative performance measures, the average minimal distance to the critical path points was computed. These points were all considered the ground-truth termination points, as it was difficult to assess which of them led

Table 1. Distance of computed propagation path from critical points, i.e. ablation, termination and circuit entrainment points marked in CARTO, i.e. critical CARTO points; characteristics of the tachycardia termination point classifier and distance of the point with the highest computed probability of termination from actual CARTO critical points.

	RV	RA	LA	TCPC	Mean
Mean distance to CARTO points [mm]	22.25	14.09	13.98	3.77	16.36
Standard deviation [mm]	13.05	12.16	6.98	3.53	12.03
Accuracy [%]	59.26	71.59	72.37	79.10	68.49
Specificity [%]	62.07	75.64	75.40	82.26	71.94
Sensitivity [%]	38.54	33.06	47.62	40.00	37.52
Avg. min. dist. to CARTO points [mm]	0.00	2.84	0.00	2.46	1.52
Standard deviation [mm]	0.00	4.19	0.00	0.00	3.06

to the tachycardia termination. For every path point, the closest critical path point was found. This distance was then averaged over all path points.

The leave-one-out ensemble learning yielded a mean accuracy of 68.49 % in detecting critical points along the propagation path (Table 1). The points with a termination probability over 50 % lay within 1.52 mm from their closest critical path point. The lowest error was recorded in RV and LA, for which all computed termination points matched a ground-truth critical point (0.00 entries in the table). The computed tachycardia termination was colour-coded to emphasize the points of highest probability. Table 1 averages the results of both circuit reconstruction and critical point detection for each type of cardiac chamber.

3.3 Performance on Subsampled Electroanatomical Maps

The path reconstruction and termination point detection algorithms were applied on 5 iterations of subsampling in each study. Results for a right atrium are presented in Table 2 which shows how the tachycardia circuit was re-shaped with the addition of new mapping points and how the classification algorithm changed its output.

4   Discussion and Conclusion

In this paper, a traversed graph representation for sparse encoding of macro-reentrant tachycardia was presented. In addition to good qualitative correlation with the geodesics in the LAT map, the Cartesian distance to the true termination and circuit entrainment points also support the applicability of the algorithm. The observed error in this study was primarily caused by the interpolation limitations in CARTO, a system error which could be alleviated with the use of another electroanatomical mapping system or in a simulated cardiac activation software.

Table 2. Sequence of propagation path reconstruction for the right atrium in Fig. 1 (upper table) and average over all cases (lower table). The points were added in decreasing order of their k-mean cluster centroid's marginal information value. A – accuracy [%], Sp – specificity [%], Se – sensitivity [%], d – minimal distance to CARTO ablation [mm], D – average distance to CARTO critical points, assumed on the ground-truth path [mm], σ – standard deviation of the distances to CARTO critical points [mm].

	Iteration #1	Iteration #2	Iteration #3	Iteration #4	Iteration #5
LAT					
Termination					
D	52.81	2.78	11.12	3.85	6.71
σ	7.67	5.17	5.17	5.17	6.71
A	73.33	42.22	50.63	35.21	60.27
Sp	78.57	37.84	50.00	37.50	62.69
Se	0.00	62.50	60.00	14.29	33.33
d	52.12	0.00	2.22	0.00	3.59

● computed path   ● ablation points   ○ circuit entrainment   ○ tachycardia termination

	Iteration #1	Iteration #2	Iteration #3	Iteration #4	Iteration #5
D	20.35	8.63	14.09	13.91	10.73
σ	17.74	7.31	7.28	9.22	7.50
A	47.71	50.96	56.68	53.99	61.82
Sp	46.93	50.09	57.91	55.32	64.59
Se	45.64	51.86	49.87	43.53	35.77
d	15.56	4.53	9.69	8.61	8.25

Also, partial anatomical maps, due to the cardiologist's interest in one particular area, lead to incompleteness of the activation wave. While constructing a more detailed map would be time consuming, operator input, where the cardiologist can correct or add features locally, is a feasible solution for better results. In this regard, the subsampling algorithm and the application of the presented method to sparse data provide guidance for the cardiologist in deciding which region needs more detailed information for a more accurate reconstruction.

In terms of termination point detection, while part of the error can be traced back to the path reconstruction inaccuracy, the learning feature vector itself can be enhanced with information such as wall thickness and estimated catheter tip motion at each point on the path, as described by [10]. The importance of additional information can be inferred from Table 2, where it is shown how different activation paths led to different termination points. Starting with only a fifth of the full set of mapping points, the detection algorithm had limited electrical data gradients to differentiate between ablation and regular sites (high sensitivity and low specificity). With the addition of mapping points, the specificity increased.

Despite the expected benefit of the leave-one-out learning of tachycardia termination, the results in Table 1 do not support this method. The most numerous cohort of RA tachycardias does not have a high score in any of the accuracy, sensitivity, or specificity. This is probably due to the high variability in the set, but also because of the error in the first stage of path reconstruction. In fact, it can be inferred from Table 1 that the termination accuracy is inversely correlated with the mean distance to the CARTO points on the ground-truth path, i.e. the path reconstruction accuracy. This is also the reason why the single TCPC case, with a small error of path reconstruction, has the best accuracy and specificity result, despite not being able to learn from other TCPC maps.

On the computational side, the two-step method of reconstruction and learning can be easily integrated into a real-time solution. The tachycardia circuit detection runs in approximately 42.2 ms. The subject-specific RUSBoost classification runs in approximately 2.1 s, considering that the data base of the training model can be learned offline and only the test data needs to be labelled. Times were measured on an i7 CPU at 2.4 GHz with unoptimised Matlab code.

In conclusion, this paper presents a method for effective combination of graph traverse and ensemble learning classification algorithms for reconstructing macro-reentrant tachycardia circuits and identifying the site of most probable termination. It is based on the identification of the shortest path from the earliest to the latest activation time along the arrhythmia propagation curve. The anatomy was modelled as a graph with edges weighted by the propagation speed between two adjacent vertices and the conductivity of the tissue measured as local potential. After reconstructing the activation path, the point of most probable termination was sought. RUSBoost was applied in a leave-one-out ensemble learning framework, where the pattern of LAT-bipolar-unipolar voltage of typical termination points was learned.

Finally, both the activation reconstruction and the termination point detection were run on subsets of the original mapping points. This anticipates re-mapping guidance after ablation in order to verify the uninducibility of the ablated tachycardia. Moreover, the reconstruction from undersampled data can provide an optimal order of mapping points acquisition in similar anatomy.

References

1. Relan, J., Chinchapatnam, P., Sermesant, M., et al.: Coupled personalization of cardiac electrophysiology models for prediction of ischaemic ventricular tachycardia. Interface Focus **1**(3), 396–407 (2011)
2. Prakosa, A., Sermesant, M., Allain, P., et al.: Cardiac electrophysiological activation pattern estimation from images using a patient-specific database of synthetic image sequences. TBME **61**(2), 235–245 (2014)

3. Mitchell, C., Schaeffer, D.: A two-current model for the dynamics of cardiac membrane. Bull. Mat. Biol. **65**, 767–793 (2003)
4. Zettinig, O., et al.: Fast data-driven calibration of a cardiac electrophysiology model from images and ECG. In: Mori, K., Sakuma, I., Sato, Y., Barillot, C., Navab, N. (eds.) MICCAI 2013, Part I. LNCS, vol. 8149, pp. 1–8. Springer, Heidelberg (2013)
5. Zhu, H., Sun, Y., Rajagopal, G., Mondry, A., Dhar, P.: Facilitating arrhythmia simulation: the method of quantitative cellular automata modeling and parallel running. Biomed. Eng. Online **3**, 29 (2004). doi:10.1186/1475-925X-3-29
6. Cárdenes, R., Sebastian, R., Soto-Iglesias, D., Andreu, D., Fernández-Armenta, J., Bijnens, B., Berruezo, A., Camara, O.: Estimation of electrical pathways finding minimal cost paths from electro-anatomical mapping of the left ventricle. In: Camara, O., Mansi, T., Pop, M., Rhode, K., Sermesant, M., Young, A. (eds.) STACOM 2013. LNCS, vol. 8330, pp. 220–227. Springer, Heidelberg (2014)
7. Cignoni, P., Corsini, M., Ranzuglia, G.: MeshLab: an open-source 3D mesh processing system. ERCIM News **73**, 45–46 (2008)
8. Dijkstra, E.: A note on two problems in connexion with graphs. Numerische Mathematik **1**, 269–271 (1959)
9. Seiffert, C., Khoshgoftaar, T., Van Hulse, J., Napolitano, A.: RUSBoost: a hybrid approach to alleviating class imbalance. Trans. Syst. Man Cybern., Part A **40**(1), 185–197 (2010)
10. Constantinescu, M., Lee, S.-L., Ernst, S., Yang, G.-Z.: Multi-source motion decoupling ablation catheter guidance for electrophysiology procedures. In: Camara, O., Mansi, T., Pop, M., Rhode, K., Sermesant, M., Young, A. (eds.) STACOM 2014. LNCS, vol. 8896, pp. 213–220. Springer, Heidelberg (2015)

Prediction of Infarct Localization from Myocardial Deformation

Nicolas Duchateau$^{(\boxtimes)}$ and Maxime Sermesant

Asclepios Research Project, INRIA, Sophia Antipolis, France
nicolas.duchateau@inria.fr

Abstract. We propose a novel framework to predict the location of a myocardial infarct from local wall deformation data. Non-linear dimensionality reduction is used to estimate the Euclidean space of coordinates encoding deformation patterns. The infarct location of a new subject is inferred by two consecutive interpolations, formulated as multiscale kernel regressions. They consist in (i) finding the low-dimensional coordinates associated to the measured deformation pattern, and (ii) estimating the possible infarct location associated to these coordinates. These concepts were tested on a database of 500 synthetic cases generated from a realistic electromechanical model of the two ventricles. The database consisted of infarcts of random extent, shape, and location overlapping the whole left-anterior-descending coronary territory. We demonstrate that our method is accurate and significantly overcomes the limitations of the clinically-used thresholding of the deformation patterns (average area under the ROC curve of 0.992±0.011 vs. 0.812±0.124, p<0.001).

1 Introduction

In clinical routine, imaging of the heart often aims at evaluating the local cardiac tissue viability. A decrease in this viability directly affects the electrical propagation and the muscle contraction, and therefore hampers the resulting cardiac function. However, the transfer function linking the local deformation to the tissue viability is complex, due to advanced physiological interactions between the muscle and the blood, the fibers arrangement, or the influence of the neighboring segments or the opposite wall. Late-enhancement imaging is generally accepted as ground truth to localize the regions with scarred tissue [8,9]. However, this modality is costly and requires the injection of a contrast agent. Moreover its post-processing is still challenging due to the limited contrast and number of acquired slices. On the other hand, 3D echocardiography is non-ionizing and cheaper, and allows the quantification of local wall deformation (myocardial strain). Cardiologists use it in a daily practice to assess the local tissue viability. Nonetheless, the localization of infarct by thresholding deformation patterns [9] is inaccurate, as the optimal threshold depends on the infarct position and grade, and the relationship between these two parameters is not straightforward.

© Springer International Publishing Switzerland 2016
O. Camara et al. (Eds.): STACOM 2015, LNCS 9534, pp. 51–59, 2016.
DOI: 10.1007/978-3-319-28712-6_6

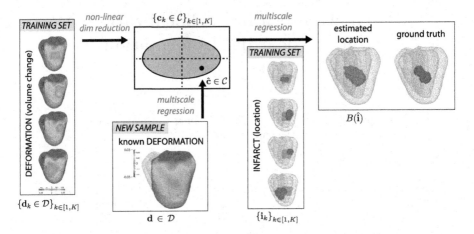

Fig. 1. Proposed method to predict infarct location from local myocardial deformation.

In this paper, we address this issue by proposing a framework to predict the infarct location from local wall deformation data. While the literature abounds of works that threshold the deformation data, our work is novel in designing a more advanced and accurate prediction strategy. Several works investigated variables inference for different cardiac applications, such as the reconstruction of fibers architecture from cardiac shape [5] or to relate cardiac shape remodeling and myocardial infarction [12]. However, these works used linear or logistic regression techniques, which are not necessarily suited to compute statistics on cardiac motion and deformation patterns. For our concrete application, we preferred a formulation based on spectral embedding [11] and kernel regression [3,4] against a Bayesian formulation, in order to minimize the amount of a-priori knowledge in our method.

A notable asset of the proposed work consists in the large database of synthetic cases created to test the methods against a large variety of infarct configurations. Indeed, in such a framework, the transfer function between the model parameters of healthy/damaged tissue and the local deformation is fully controlled, a requisite to test the methods accuracy on ground truth data. Our experiments show that the prediction of infarct location with our method is significantly more accurate than the clinically-used techniques.

2   Methods

In the following, we denote $\{(\mathbf{d}_k, \mathbf{i}_k)\}_{k\in[1,K]}$ the pairs of local deformation and infarct position data for the set of K training samples. This information is available at each point of the volumetric mesh for each subject, and each of these two parameters is treated as a column vector. In the present work, the infarct position is defined as a binary value 0/1 at each vertex. The relative change in the cell volume with respect to the beginning of the cycle is used as a surrogate for local deformation. A single scalar value is therefore associated to the deformation at each point of the mesh. This was preferred over more advanced measures of local deformation such as the strain tensor, which would require more advanced statistics. However, using scalar deformation data does not limit the concepts demonstrated in the present work: the observed deformation patterns still reflect local infarct (Figs. 1 and 4), and focus is kept on the core of the inverse problem.

2.1 Non-linear Dimensionality Reduction (Training Set)

The (high-dimensional) local deformation data $\{\mathbf{d}_k \in \mathcal{D}\}_{k \in [1,K]}$ are first mapped to a Euclidean space of (low-dimensional) coordinates $\{\mathbf{c}_k \in \mathcal{C}\}_{k \in [1,K]}$ by means of standard non-linear dimensionality reduction (Isomap [10]). This assumes that there exists a lower-dimensional manifold that can explain the main variations in such data.

In brief, a nearest-neighbors graph is built for the samples $\{\mathbf{d}_k\}_{k \in [1,K]}$, using the Euclidean distance as metric. Then, the geodesic distance between each pair of samples is approximated as the shortest path connecting them along the graph, and put into an affinity matrix. The set of coordinates $\{\mathbf{c}_k\}_{k \in [1,K]}$ is finally obtained by the diagonalization of a centered version of this geodesic distance matrix.

No restriction is made on the manifold learning technique used. We preferred a non-linear one, as linear operations directly on the deformation data may generate unphysiological patterns [2,4] (e.g. the linear average of two deformation patterns corresponding to two disjoint infarcts would provide a mixed widespread pattern reflecting a larger but less accentuated infarct, instead of the pattern of an infarct of similar grade at an intermediate location). The Isomap algorithm was preferred over other spectral embedding techniques [11] as we assumed that the samples distribution follows a uniform random distribution, in contrast with kernel-based methods more relevant for more clustered distributions.

2.2 From Deformation Patterns to Infarct Prediction (Testing Set)

Given a new case for which only the local deformation $\mathbf{d}$ is known, our method provides a prediction of the infarct position $B(\hat{\mathbf{i}})$. Its estimation is obtained by two consecutive interpolations formulated as kernel regression, and a multiscale strategy to prevent from artifacts due to non-uniformities in the density of the samples. An overview of the processing pipeline is given in Fig. 1.

From Deformation Patterns to Low-Dimensional Coordinates. Given a new deformation pattern $\mathbf{d} \in \mathcal{D}$, a single-scale formulation would compute its corresponding coordinates $\hat{\mathbf{c}} \in \mathcal{C}$ as:

$$\hat{\mathbf{c}} = \sum_{k=1}^{K} k_{\mathcal{D}}(\mathbf{d}, \mathbf{d}_k) \cdot \mathbf{a}_k. \tag{1}$$

Here $\mathbf{a}_k$ is the k-th column of the matrix $(\mathbf{K}_{\mathcal{D}} + \frac{1}{\gamma_{\mathcal{D}}}\mathbf{I})^{-1}\mathbb{C}$, where $\mathbf{I}$ is the identity matrix, $\mathbb{C} = (\mathbf{c}_1, \ldots, \mathbf{c}_K)^T$, $\gamma_{\mathcal{D}}$ is a scalar weight balancing the adherence to the data and the smoothness of the interpolation, and $\mathbf{K}_{\mathcal{D}} = (k_{\mathcal{D}}(\mathbf{d}_i, \mathbf{d}_j))_{(i,j)}$ is a kernel-based affinity matrix between the input samples. The kernel function is defined as $k_{\mathcal{D}} = \exp(-\|\mathbf{d}_i - \mathbf{d}_j\|^2 / \sigma_{\mathcal{D}}^2)$, $\sigma_{\mathcal{D}}$ being its bandwidth.

Detailed explanations of this single-scale process can be found in [2]. The expression in Eq. 1 corresponds to the analytical solution of the following inexact matching problem:

$$\underset{\tilde{f} \in \mathcal{F}}{\operatorname{argmin}} \left(\frac{1}{2} \|f\|_{\mathcal{F}}^2 + \frac{\gamma_{\mathcal{D}}}{2} \sum_{k=1}^{K} \|f(\mathbf{d}_k) - \mathbf{c}_k\|^2 \right), \qquad (2)$$

where $\hat{\mathbf{c}} = f(\mathbf{d})$, and $\|.\|_{\mathcal{F}}$ stands for the norm on the reproducible kernel Hilbert space $\mathcal{F}$ of functions $\mathcal{D} \to \mathcal{C}$.

In the current application, this process is iterated from large to small scales by dividing the bandwidth $\sigma_{\mathcal{D}}$ by a factor 2 at each iteration s, and looking for the remainder function $f - F^{(s-1)}$, where $F^{(s)}$ stands for the s-th scale approximation of the original function f [3]. In practice, scales across iterations range from the overall spread of the samples until getting lower than the average density of the samples [3].

From Low-Dimensional Coordinates to Infarct Prediction. An infarct map $\hat{\mathbf{i}} \in \mathcal{I}$ is estimated from the coordinates $\hat{\mathbf{c}}$ using a multiscale regression process similar to the one described in the previous subsection, where $\hat{\mathbf{i}}$, $\hat{\mathbf{c}}$ and $\mathbf{c}_k$ now respectively stand for $\hat{\mathbf{c}}$, $\mathbf{d}$ and $\mathbf{d}_k$ in Eq. 1. The interpolating function is now denoted g. The infarct map therefore corresponds to $\hat{\mathbf{i}} = g(\hat{\mathbf{c}}) = g \circ f(\mathbf{d})$. Data adherence and smoothness are balanced by a weight $\gamma_{\mathcal{C}}$, and the kernel function is $k_{\mathcal{C}}$, of bandwidth $\sigma_{\mathcal{C}}$. In a single-scale formulation, this corresponds to:

$$\hat{\mathbf{i}} = \sum_{k=1}^{K} k_{\mathcal{C}}(\hat{\mathbf{c}}, \mathbf{c}_k) \cdot \mathbf{b}_k, \qquad (3)$$

where $\mathbf{b}_k$ is the k-th column of the matrix $(\mathbf{K}_{\mathcal{C}} + \frac{1}{\gamma_{\mathcal{C}}}\mathbb{I})^{-1}\mathbb{I}$, $\mathbb{I} = (\mathbf{i}_1, \ldots, \mathbf{i}_K)^T$, and $\mathbf{K}_{\mathcal{C}} = (k_{\mathcal{C}}(\mathbf{c}_i, \mathbf{c}_j))_{(i,j)}$. This process is also made multiscale, and follows similar rules to the ones used for the estimation of f.

Due to this regression process, the values of $\hat{\mathbf{i}}$ at each vertex lie within the continuous $[0, 1]$ interval. Thus, the prediction of the infarct position $B(\hat{\mathbf{i}})$ is finally obtained by applying a relevant threshold to $\hat{\mathbf{i}}$ (in our case, previously determined by a ROC analysis, as described in Sect. 3.2).

3   Experiments and Results

3.1   Dataset

Infarct Generation. A database of 500 synthetic cases was generated to evaluate the methods. Starting from a volumetric tetrahedral mesh of the two ventricles (46876 cells and 9673 points for the left ventricle [LV], corresponding to a

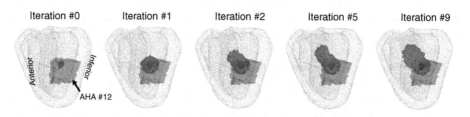

Fig. 2. Iterative generation of an infarcted region (*red*) with random extent, shape, and location, initiated within the mid-anterolateral segment (*black arrow*) (Color figure online).

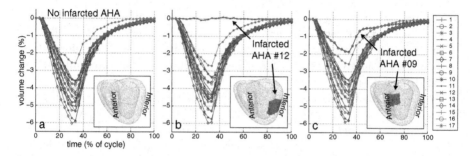

Fig. 3. Average myocardial deformation for each AHA segment in a healthy case (*a*), and two infarcts in opposite AHA segments (*b* and *c*).

myocardial volume/mass of 173 mL/182 g), a fully-connected region corresponding to an infarct of random extent, shape, and location was constructed for each case. The algorithm determined the diseased region iteratively, as illustrated in Fig. 2. It first randomly selected a starting point within the left-anterior-descending coronary territory. This specific territory was retained due to its higher prevalence and agreement in its delineation [8]. Note that this only concerns the location of the starting point for the infarct generation algorithm, and that infarcts can spread out of this territory (Fig. 4). Further testing should be extended to other coronary territories and different geometries to better evaluate the performance of the method.

A spherical neighborhood of random radius between 2 and 12 mm was marked as diseased, and a new starting point was randomly selected within this new region. The process was iterated a random number of times (values from 1 to 16). Infarct extents were of 5.2±2.6 mL (3.0±1.5 % of the LV myocardium). A total of 400 cases were used as training set and the other 100 served as testing data.

Electromechanical Simulation. A realistic electromechanical model [6] was then used to simulate the cardiac function along a full cycle of duration 1 s. This model was previously evaluated on invasive clinical data and has a realistic behavior. Simulations here use a real anatomical mesh with fibers architecture from an atlas. The contractility and stiffness parameters were altered in the random zone defined by our algorithm to model a local infarct [1]. They partially reflect changes in active force and tissue elasticity. These parameters were retained among many others to limit the training data to manageable amounts, and corresponded to the ones with major influence on the deformation [7]. Border zone was not set to only evaluate the algorithm on binary prediction. Neighbor locations were therefore only passively influenced by the infarct.

Then, local deformation was computed for each tetrahedral cell of the mesh. Figure 3 depicts the deformation values of two infarct configurations at opposite AHA segments, against a healthy case. In this illustrative example, the whole AHA segment was infarcted. Curves represent volume change values averaged over each of the 17 AHA segments of the LV. Notably, deformation patterns are less affected by a mid-anterolateral infarct than by a mid-inferoseptal one, due to the influence of the right ventricle and the surrounding septal regions. Testing our methods on a wide territory of infarct configurations will therefore allow evaluating the sensitivity of the algorithm to marked or moderate alterations of local deformation.

For the sake of simplicity in the infarct prediction process, we limited the input to our algorithm to the deformation data at end-systole (the $\{\mathbf{d}_k \in \mathcal{D}\}_{k \in [1,K]}$ in Sect. 2), spatially smoothed by a Gaussian filter of bandwidth 1 cm to prevent from inconsistencies due to point-cell correspondences and the non-homogeneity of cell sizes and orientation across the whole volumetric mesh. Note that this might lower the accuracy of the infarct prediction near the border of the ground truth location. The use of the deformation data along the whole cycle may add robustness to the results in more complex configurations, where local post-systolic abnormalities may be more marked or in the presence of asynchronous hearts.

Parameters Setting. The number of nearest neighbors in the Isomap algorithm was set to 5. The number of dimensions retained for the estimated coordinates was set to 30. This value corresponded to the limit from which eigenvalues weigh less than 5 % of the first eigenvalue. The scalar weights used in the multiscale regression were determined by a leave-one-out procedure, as the value that minimizes the generalization ability (the reconstruction error for samples lying within the range of noise of the training set). Such values were of $\gamma_\mathcal{D} = \gamma_\mathcal{C} = 1$.

3.2 Results

Representative examples of the outputs of our method are shown in Fig. 4, to compare with the thresholding of the deformation data from the same cases, in Fig. 5 (animated version available as *Supplementary Material*[1]). The latter notably failed on the transmurality of the infarct location. Qualitatively, our method correctly predicted the infarct location, even for infarcts of small size, location internal to the myocardium, and reduced effect on the deformation curves (e.g. infarcts closer to the septum).

---

[1] http://www-sop.inria.fr/asclepios/docs/TestCasesThresh.zip.

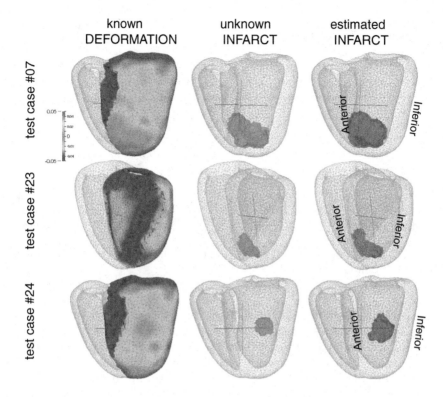

Fig. 4. Examples of myocardial deformation pattern, ground truth infarct location, and estimated infarct location (Color figure online).

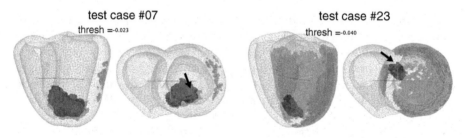

Fig. 5. Ground truth infarct location (*red*) against the thresholding of the deformation patterns (*blue*) for the cases shown in Fig. 4. Animated version available as *Supplementary Material* (see footnote 1).

ROC Analysis. On each case, a ROC analysis was used to determine the optimal threshold leading to the infarct prediction $B(\hat{\mathbf{i}})$ from the infarct map $\hat{\mathbf{i}} \in \mathcal{I}$ (Fig. 6a). A similar process was applied for the direct thresholding of the deformation data $\mathbf{d} \in \mathcal{D}$ (Fig. 6b). These thresholds were defined as the average of the optimal thresholds for each individual case.

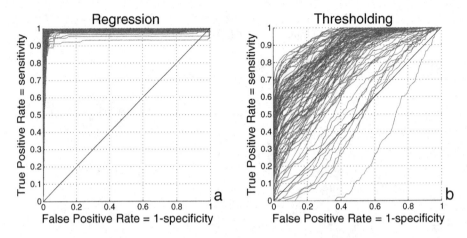

Fig. 6. ROC analysis of the tested cases comparing our method (*a*) to the thresholding of the deformation patterns (*b*).

The performance of directly thresholding the deformation was rather poor in terms of sensitivity and specificity (average area under the curve: 0.812 ± 0.124). Some cases even led to a ROC curve worse than randomly selecting points of the mesh (the diagonal line). Our method significantly outperformed this technique in all cases (average area under the curve: 0.992 ± 0.011, $p < 0.001$).

4   Conclusion

We presented a method to predict the location of a myocardial infarct from local deformation patterns. This approach is novel and contrasts with the simpler and clinically-used thresholding of the deformation patterns. Notably, our method significantly outperformed this technique. A notable asset of the proposed work also resides in the large database used to test the methods, made of synthetic cases with infarcts of random extent, shape, and location. We are currently collecting a database of 3D echocardiographic sequences and late-enhancement images to extend the evaluation of our method to real data. This will allow evaluating the scalability of the method towards the use of different heart geometries, more complex deformation patterns, and possibly less contrasted local changes in the deformation data to the acquisition and post-processing of ultrasound sequences.

Acknowledgements. The authors acknowledge the European Union 7th Framework Programme (VP2HF: FP7-2013-611823) and the European Research Council (MedYMA: ERC-AdG-2011-291080). They also thank their colleagues R. Mollero and S. Giffard-Roisin for their support on practical aspects of the SOFA simulations, and their collaborators M. De Craene (Philips Suresnes, France) and E. Saloux (CHU Caen, France) for discussions on these concepts.

References

1. Alessandrini, M., De Craene, M., Bernard, O., et al.: A pipeline for the generation of realistic 3D synthetic echocardiographic sequences: methodology and open-access database. IEEE Trans. Med. Imaging (in press, 2015)

2. Duchateau, N., De Craene, M., Piella, G., et al.: Constrained manifold learning for the characterization of pathological deviations from normality. Med. Image Anal. **16**, 1532–1549 (2012)

3. Duchateau, N., De Craene, M., Sitges, M., Caselles, V.: Adaptation of multiscale function extension to inexact matching: application to the mapping of individuals to a learnt manifold. In: Nielsen, F., Barbaresco, F. (eds.) GSI 2013. LNCS, vol. 8085, pp. 578–586. Springer, Heidelberg (2013)

4. Gerber, S., Tasdizen, T., Fletcher, P., et al.: Manifold modeling for brain population analysis. Med. Image Anal. **14**, 643–653 (2010)

5. Lekadir, K., Hoogendoorn, C., Pereanez, M., et al.: Statistical personalization of ventricular fiber orientation using shape predictors. IEEE Trans. Med. Imaging **33**, 882–890 (2014)

6. Marchesseau, S., Delingette, H., Sermesant, M., et al.: Personalization of a cardiac electromechanical model using reduced order unscented Kalman filtering from regional volumes. Med. Image Anal. **17**, 816–829 (2013)

7. Marchesseau, S., Delingette, H., Sermesant, M., Sorine, M., Rhode, K., Duckett, S., Rinaldi, C., Razavi, R., Ayache, N.: Preliminary specificity study of the Bestel-Clement-Sorine electromechanical model of the heart using parameter calibration from medical images. J. Mech. Behav. Biomed. Mater. **20**, 259–271 (2013)

8. Ortiz-Perez, J., Rodriguez, J., Meyers, S., et al.: Correspondence between the 17-segment model and coronary arterial anatomy using contrast-enhanced cardiac magnetic resonance imaging. JACC Cardiovasc. Imaging **1**, 282–292 (2008)

9. Sjøli, B., Ørn, S., Grenne, B., et al.: Diagnostic capability and reproducibility of strain by Doppler and by speckle tracking in patients with acute myocardial infarction. JACC Cardiovasc. Imaging **2**, 24–33 (2009)

10. Tenenbaum, J., De Silva, V., Langford, J.: A global geometric framework for non-linear dimensionality reduction. Science **290**, 2319–2323 (2000)

11. Yan, S., Xu, D., Zhang, B., et al.: Graph embedding and extensions: a general framework for dimensionality reduction. IEEE Trans. Pattern Anal. Mach. Intell. **29**, 40–51 (2007)

12. Zhang, X., Cowan, B., Bluemke, D., et al.: Atlas-based quantification of cardiac remodeling due to myocardial infarction. PLoS One **9**, e110243 (2014)

Parameterisation of Multi-directional Diffusion Weighted Magnetic Resonance Images of the Heart

Bianca Freytag[1]([✉]), Vicky Y. Wang[1], G. Richard Christie[1],
Alexander J. Wilson[1,2], Gregory B. Sands[1,2], Ian J. LeGrice[1,2],
Alistair A. Young[1,3], and Martyn P. Nash[1,4]

[1] Auckland Bioengineering Institute, University of Auckland, Auckland, New Zealand
{b.freytag,vicky.wang,r.christie,alexander.wilson,g.sands,i.legrice,
a.young,martyn.nash}@auckland.ac.nz
[2] Department of Physiology, University of Auckland, Auckland, New Zealand
[3] Department of Anatomy with Radiology, University of Auckland,
Auckland, New Zealand
[4] Department of Engineering Science, University of Auckland,
Auckland, New Zealand

Abstract. This study presents a novel method for building parametric representations of myocardial microstructure of the left ventricle from multi-directional diffusion weighted magnetic resonance images (DWI). The direction of maximal diffusion is directly estimated from the DWI signal intensities using finite element field fitting. This framework avoids the need to compute diffusion tensors, which introduces errors due to least squares fitting that are generally neglected when building microstructural models of the heart from DWI. Nodal parameters describing cardiac myocyte orientations throughout a finite element model of the left ventricle were fitted to a series of raw diffusion signals using non-linear least squares optimisation to determine the direction of maximum diffusion. An *ex vivo* DWI data set from a Wystar-Kyoto rat was processed using the proposed method. The fitted myocyte orientations were compared against conventional diffusion tensor/eigenvector analysis and the degree of correlation was measured using a normalised dot product (nDP). Good agreement (nDP $= 0.979$) between the new method and the traditional tensor analysis approach was observed for regions of high fractional anisotropy (FA). In regions of low FA, the errors were much more variable, but the proposed method maintains a smoothly varying myocyte angle distribution as is generally used in tissue and organ scale heart models.

Keywords: Finite element parameterisation · Cardiac myocyte orientation · Diffusion tensor magnetic resonance imaging · Raw diffusion signals

© Springer International Publishing Switzerland 2016
O. Camara et al. (Eds.): STACOM 2015, LNCS 9534, pp. 60–68, 2016.
DOI: 10.1007/978-3-319-28712-6_7

1   Introduction

Building heart models for investigating the electrical [1–3], biomechanical [4–7], and energetic function of the heart [8,9] is crucial to fully understand the underlying effects of cardiac diseases. For such heart models, finite element (FE) interpolation is generally used to describe cardiac geometry and microstructure. These models allow for integration of structural and functional data acquired using various imaging modalities, together with other measurements, such as haemodynamic or electrophysiological recordings, to analyse the electro-mechanics of the heart on a subject-specific basis.

Shape and microstructural tissue organisation are important, well-established determinants of the biomechanical function of the heart. While *in vivo* measurements of cardiac geometry are readily available via computed tomography, magnetic resonance imaging (MRI), or ultrasound, *in vivo* microstructural measurements from the whole heart remain sparse and difficult to quantify.

One option for acquiring microstructural information throughout the whole heart is to use diffusion weighted MRI (DWI). This imaging modality exploits the Brownian motion of water molecules within myocardial tissue to determine local anisotropic diffusion in the ventricular walls [10]. Several approaches have been explored to determine myocyte orientations, using either *ex vivo* or *in vivo* imaging [11–15]. Typically, a diffusion tensor is derived at each voxel from the acquired DWI, and the direction of maximum water diffusion, as represented by the primary eigenvector of the derived local diffusion tensor, has been found to correlate well with the local histologically-measured myocyte orientation [16,17]. The myocyte orientation is often represented as a helix angle with respect to the short-axis plane of the heart. FE models typically incorporate the spatial distribution of fibre orientations by interpolating helix angle parameters at the nodes of the FE mesh [2,5,6]. Representing and analysing the apparent diffusion with diffusion tensors comes with several drawbacks [18] including: (1) spatial discontinuities in helix angle distributions; and (2) misrepresentation of myocyte orientation in regions of high image noise or low fractional anisotropy (FA).

A third issue arises from the use of least squares fitting methods when calculating a diffusion tensor for each voxel. This leads to a generally neglected error, which expresses how well a tensor can represent the underlying diffusion behaviour. Figure 1(b) shows a slice extracted from the whole heart (Fig. 1(a)), indicating the coefficient of determination (R^2) of the least squares fit for each diffusion tensor[1]. If the data can be well represented by a diffusion tensor,

---

[1] The fitted diffusion tensor was projected back onto the original set of j gradient directions to get a set of estimated signal strengths ($S_{e(j)}$). The estimated signal strengths, the measured signal strengths ($S_{m(j)}$), and the mean of the measured signal strengths ($\bar{S}_m$) were then used to calculate the coefficient of determination:

$$R^2 = 1 - \frac{\sum_j (S_{m(j)} - S_{e(j)})^2}{\sum_j (S_{m(j)} - \bar{S}_m)^2}.$$ (1)

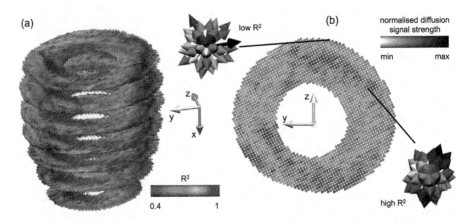

Fig. 1. Suitability of representing DWI voxels using a diffusion tensor, as indicated by the coefficient of determination (R^2) of the least squares tensor fit for (a) the whole heart and (b) one mid-ventricular slice. Normalised diffusion signals are plotted as vectors at two voxels; one with a low fitting error (high R^2) where the vectors can be well represented by an ellipsoid (diffusion tensor), and one with a high fitting error (low R^2) where the signals would be poorly represented by an ellipsoid.

the R^2 would be close to 1 and therefore the error in fitting a tensor to the data would be low. In these cases, the data show a clear apparent diffusion direction. On the other hand, the diffusion tensor can be a poor representation of the DWI data for some voxels, especially if non-adjacent directions have very high normalised signal strengths. We propose that avoiding the intermediate step of least squares fitting of a diffusion tensor would therefore be useful for understanding the accuracy of the FE field and sensitivity to variation/noise in the DWI data.

In this study we have extended the modelling framework presented in [18] to avoid the least squares error issue by direct parameterisation of the myocyte orientation field from the raw diffusion signals. In contrast to the conventional method, the intermediate step of diffusion tensor calculation is not required in this process and the raw diffusion signals are carried all the way through from image acquisition to the final fibre field fitting process.

2   Methods

2.1   Experimental Procedure

The experimental study was approved by the Animal Ethics Committee of the University of Auckland and conforms to the National Institutes of Health Guide for the Care and Use of Laboratory Animals (NIH Publication No. 85-23).

A Wistar-Kyoto rat heart was excised, perfused with St Thomas cardioplegic solution for relaxation, and fixed using Bouins solution in an approximate end-diastolic state. DWI was performed using a 3D fast spin-echo pulse sequence on a Varian 4.7 T MRI scanner. The image set consisted of 12 short-axis slices with a thickness of 1.5 mm, and no gap between slices; the in-plane resolution was set to 128 voxels × 64 voxels (zero-pad interpolated to 128 voxels × 128 voxels) with an in-plane voxel dimension of 156 μm × 156 μm. The image data for each slice contained one non-diffusion weighted anatomical image, and 30 diffusion weighted images. The 30 diffusion gradient directions were evenly distributed across a hemisphere. Further details in [18].

2.2   Workflow for Myocyte Orientation Field Parameterisation

The following method was developed to parameterise a spatially-varying myocyte orientation field for the LV myocardium directly from the raw diffusion signals (i.e. without the calculation of diffusion tensors).

Step 1: Image Segmentation and LV FE Geometric Model Construction. The endocardial and epicardial surfaces of the LV, excluding the papillary muscles, were manually segmented from the non-diffusion images using MATLAB[2]. Three landmark points (LV base, LV apex, and right ventricle (RV) base) defined the orientation of the orthogonal cardiac coordinate system (further details in [18]).

A prolate spheroidal-shaped 16-element (4 circumferential, 4 longitudinal and 1 transmural) hexahedral tri-cubic Hermite FE model was customised to the segmented surfaces to represent the LV geometry. The surfaces of the model were fitted using non-linear least squares minimisation.

Step 2: Field-Based Parameterisation of LV Myocyte Orientation. To parameterise the myocyte orientation field throughout the LV FE geometric model, we developed a novel method to estimate spatially-continuous myocyte angle fields (interpolated using tri-cubic Hermite basis functions) that best represent the maximal diffusion direction at all voxels within the LV. Firstly, the myocyte orientation field was initialised by setting the helix angles ($\theta_{(n)}$) to 0° for endocardial and epicardial nodes. Initial imbrication angles ($\varphi_{(n)}$) at all nodes were also set to 0°. Secondly, the FE local coordinates within the LV geometric model were determined for each voxel (v), and an estimate of the myocyte orientation ($\mathbf{f}_{(v)}$) at each voxel was interpolated. This was done by Euler angle rotations of vectors [19] by the interpolated angles $\theta_{(n)}$ and $\varphi_{(n)}$.

To express the amount of diffusion along the jth gradient direction ($\mathbf{g}_{(j)}$) we introduced a weight ($w_{(j,v)}$) for direction j in voxel v derived from the basic diffusion equation[3]:

$$S_{(j,v)} = S_{(0,v)}e^{-\gamma^2 G^2 D_{(j)}\delta^2(\Delta-\frac{\delta}{3})}. \tag{2}$$

---

[2] The MathWorks, Inc., Natick, Massachusetts, United States.

[3] γ represents the gyromagnetic ratio of protons, δ and G the duration and magnitude of application of the motion probing gradient along direction $\mathbf{g}_{(j)}$, $D_{(j)}$ the apparent diffusivity in the same direction, and Δ the time difference between the centres of a pair of gradient pulses.

Rearranging Eq. 2 gives:

$$- \ln\left(\frac{S_{(j,v)}}{S_{(0,v)}}\right) = \gamma^2 G^2 D_{(j)} \delta^2 \left(\Delta - \frac{\delta}{3}\right) \equiv w_{(j,v)}. \tag{3}$$

Scaling the unit vectors $\mathbf{g}_{(j)}$ by $w_{(j,v)}$ provided weighted direction vectors $(\mathbf{w}_{(j,v)})$ that represented the magnitude of diffusion along each gradient direction. Finally, an objective function (Ψ) was constructed:

$$\Psi = \sum_v \sum_j (\mathbf{w}_{(j,v)} \cdot \mathbf{f}_{(v)})^2, \tag{4}$$

which is greatest when $\mathbf{f}_{(v)}$ is aligned with the directions of $\mathbf{w}_{(j,v)}$ with greatest magnitude. The objective function was maximised using non-linear optimisation[4] by modifying the nodal parameters ($\theta_{(n)}$ and $\varphi_{(n)}$). The method was implemented using the OpenCMISS-Cmgui software package[5] [20].

2.3   Surrogate Estimate of Fractional Anisotropy

By avoiding the calculation of a diffusion tensor the conventional estimate of FA from the eigenvalues of the diffusion tensor is not available. FA describes how much the ellipsoid associated with a diffusion tensor differs from a sphere. To provide an equivalent index, we derived an estimate of FA from the raw diffusion signals (rdsFA) in a formulation similar to the expression used to compute FA from the eigenvalues of the diffusion tensor [21]:

$$\text{rdsFA} = \sqrt{\frac{d}{d-1} \frac{\sum_j (w_{(j)} - \bar{w})^2}{\sum_j w_{(j)}^2}}, \tag{5}$$

where d is the number of directions and

$$\bar{w} = \frac{1}{d} \sum_j w_{(j)}. \tag{6}$$

This enabled a comparison of the relative anisotropy between voxels without the need to compute diffusion tensors. As a comparison with the conventional approach, we found that there was a strong linear correlation between FA and rdsFA (correlation coefficient of $R^2 = 0.9975$).

3   Results

Having fitted the myocyte orientation field to the raw diffusion signals, the myocyte angles were then interpolated at each of the image voxel locations. The

---

[4] least squares quasi Newton function, OPT++ optimisation library, http://software. sandia.gov/opt++.

[5] OpenCMISS-Cmgui application, www.opencmiss.org.

result is plotted in Fig. 2(a) using the helix angle to colour-code the myocyte orientation. The helix angle field varied smoothly throughout the LV, with positive angles at the endocardium and negative angles at the epicardial surface.

We compared the fitted myocyte orientations ($\mathbf{f}_{(v)}$) with the primary eigenvectors ($\mathbf{e}_{1(v)}$) calculated by conventional eigenanalysis of the diffusion tensors. We used a normalised dot product (nDP, see Eq. 7) to quantify the overall alignment of the fitted orientation and the primary eigenvector at each voxel by scaling their dot product by the $FA_{(v)}$ at the corresponding voxel. This accounts for the differing degree of confidence in the calculated eigenvectors since a voxel with a FA of 0 does not have a unique primary eigenvector. nDP ranges from 0 to 1, with 1 representing a perfect alignment of both vectors within an image voxel. The resulting nDP in this study was very close to 1, which suggests a high correlation between the primary eigenvector of the diffusion tensor and the fitted myocyte orientation across all myocardial voxels:

$$\text{nDP} = \frac{\sum_v (FA_{(v)} |\mathbf{f}_{(v)} \cdot \mathbf{e}_{1(v)}|)}{\sum_v FA_{(v)}} = 0.979. \tag{7}$$

When building personalised models of the heart based on primary eigenvectors of diffusion tensors, it is common to parameterise myocyte orientations using a FE model by interpolating their spatial distribution (after phase-unwrapping). We processed the primary eigenvectors with this approach to provide a comparison set of myocyte orientations ($\mathbf{h}_{(v)}$) fitted to the eigenvectors $\mathbf{e}_{1(v)}$.

Figure 2(b) presents a map of FA (top) in a mid-ventricular slice, along with the alignment between $\mathbf{f}_{(v)}$ and $\mathbf{e}_{1(v)}$ (bottom-left), and between $\mathbf{f}_{(v)}$ and $\mathbf{h}_{(v)}$ (bottom-right). At locations where FA was high, the directions were similar, however significant differences were observed in regions of low FA (highlighted with dashed boxes in Fig. 2(b)). The alignment with spatially-interpolated eigenvectors was much closer, and remaining differences, which tended to arise near boundaries, may have been caused by those voxels containing partial-volume imaging artefacts.

Figure 3 shows transmural gradients of raw and fitted helix angles at two locations around the LV wall, and illustrates that even in regions of low FA, such as the intersection of LV and RV, this method provided a smoothly varying myocyte angle field.

4   Discussion

A novel method was developed to parameterise a continuous myocyte orientation field throughout a FE model of the LV by directly fitting to raw diffusion signals acquired by DWI. This method circumvents issues associated with the eigenanalysis of diffusion tensors that can potentially lead to misrepresentation of the local myocyte orientation. These disadvantages can have a significant impact on electrophysiological and mechanical modelling studies as they affect the description of the electrical, contractile, and passive mechanical constitutive properties of the tissue. In addition, this new method does not assume the diffusion to be

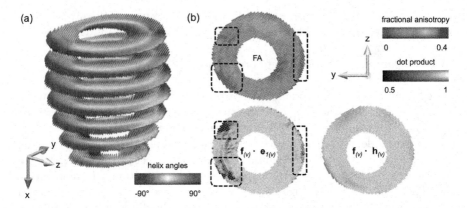

Fig. 2. (a) Fitted myocyte orientations colour-coded by the interpolated helix angles at all voxels within the LV. (b) A mid-ventricular slice showing (top) FA, and the alignment between interpolated myocyte orientations $\mathbf{f}_{(v)}$ and (bottom-left) primary eigenvectors $\mathbf{e}_{1(v)}$, and (bottom-right) between $\mathbf{f}_{(v)}$ and spatially-interpolated eigenvectors $\mathbf{h}_{(v)}$. The dotted squares indicate (top) areas of low FA and (bottom) corresponding regions of poor alignment. The FA spectrum was set to range between 0 and 0.4 to highlight the regional variability (Color figure online).

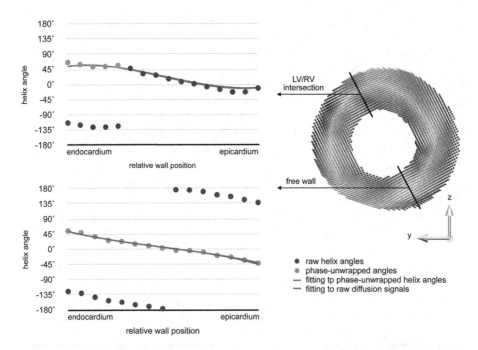

Fig. 3. Transmural gradients of helix angle along the indicated lines at the intersection of LV and RV and at the LV free wall. Fitting to the raw diffusion signals (red lines) shows good agreement with the raw helix angles. The result for fitting to the helix angles is illustrated for comparison reasons (Color figure online).

best represented by a tensor, and thus avoids the loss of information associated with the least squares fit of the diffusion tensor. Instead of using a voxel-wise data reduction to a tensor, the new method incorporates the spatial distribution of diffusion signals. The error therefore only involves one fitting process instead of two by eliminating the intermediate step of least squares fitting of the diffusion tensor, and requires less computation. It would be possible to further extend this technique to capture microstructural features that are not well represented by a diffusion tensor. One example would be to represent crossing fibres by allowing multiple orientations within a single voxel, and another would be to allow the representation of tissue isotropy (where there is no preferred direction) as it may be found in regions of myocyte disarray. Myocyte orientations estimated using this method agree well with the conventional method of fitting a myocyte field to primary eigenvectors for regions of high FA, within which the primary eigenvector has been shown to reliably represent the local myocyte orientation. In regions of low FA, this method provides continuously varying myocyte orientations. If the main contributor to low FA is noise, then maintaining continuity in the myocyte orientation field despite low FA is an important advantage.

The results suggest that fitting to the raw diffusion signals gives a better representation of the underlying structure than fitting to the primary eigenvectors of diffusion tensors, because the objective function implicitly accounts for variations in FA.

5 Conclusions

In this study, a model-based parameterisation method was proposed to directly interpret diffusion signals provided by *ex vivo* DWI. Our scheme does not require the conventional calculation of diffusion tensors, but directly fits a myocyte orientation field to spatial distributions of raw diffusion signals. A comparison of the proposed framework with a conventional eigenvector fitting method showed good agreement in regions of high FA, and smooth solutions in regions with low FA. Future studies will include exploring the influence of noise and motion artefacts on the fitting results.

References

1. Vadakkumpadan, F., Gurev, V., Constantino, J., Arevalo, H., Trayanova, N.: Modeling of whole-heart electrophysiology and mechanics: toward patient-specific simulations. In: Kerckhoff, R.C.P. (ed.) Patient-Specific Modeling of the Cardiovascular System, pp. 145–165. Springer, New York (2010)
2. Sermesant, M., Chabiniok, R., et al.: Patient-specific electromechanical models of the heart for the prediction of pacing acute effects in CRT: a preliminary clinical validation. Med. Image Anal. 16(1), 201–215 (2012)
3. Keldermann, R.H., Nash, M.P., Gelderblom, H., Wang, V.Y., Panfilov, A.V.: Electromechanical wavebreak in a model of the human left ventricle. Am. J. Physiol. Heart Circulatory Physiol. 299(1), H134–H143 (2010)
4. Krishnamurthy, A., Villongco, C.T., et al.: Patient-specific models of cardiac biomechanics. J. Comput. Phys. 244, 4–21 (2013)

5. Walker, J.C., Ratcliffe, M.B., Zhang, P., Wallace, A.W., Hsu, E.W., Saloner, D.A., Guccione, J.M.: Magnetic resonance imaging-based finite element stress analysis after linear repair of left ventricular aneurysm. J. Thoracic Cardiovasc. Surg. **135**(5), 1094–1102 (2008)
6. Wang, V.Y., Lam, H., Ennis, D.B., Cowan, B.R., Young, A.A., Nash, M.P.: Modelling passive diastolic mechanics with quantitative MRI of cardiac structure and function. Med. Image Anal. **13**(5), 773–784 (2009)
7. Xi, J., Lamata, P., et al.: The estimation of patient-specific cardiac diastolic functions from clinical measurements. Med. Image Anal. **17**(2), 133–146 (2013)
8. Niederer, S.A., Smith, N.P.: The role of the frank-starling law in the transduction of cellular work to whole organ pump function: a computational modeling analysis. PLoS Comput. Biol. **5**(4), e1000371 (2009)
9. Wang, V.Y., Ennis, D.B., Cowan, B.R., Young, A.A., Nash, M.P.: Myocardial contractility and regional work throughout the cardiac cycle using FEM and MRI. In: Camara, O., Konukoglu, E., Pop, M., Rhode, K., Sermesant, M., Young, A. (eds.) STACOM 2011. LNCS, vol. 7085, pp. 149–159. Springer, Heidelberg (2012)
10. Basser, P.J., Mattiello, J., LeBihan, D.: Estimation of the effective self-diffusion tensor from the NMR spin echo. J. Magn. Reson. Series B **103**(3), 247–254 (1994)
11. Lekadir, K., Hoogendoorn, C., Pereanez, M., Albà, X., Pashaei, A., Frangi, A.F.: Statistical personalization of ventricular fiber orientation using shape predictors. IEEE Trans. Med. Imaging **33**(4), 882–890 (2014)
12. Toussaint, N., Stoeck, C.T., Schaeffter, T., Kozerke, S., Sermesant, M., Batchelor, P.G.: In vivo human cardiac fibre architecture estimation using shape-based diffusion tensor processing. Med. Image Anal. **17**(8), 1243–1255 (2013)
13. Jones, D.K., Pierpaoli, C.: Confidence mapping in diffusion tensor magnetic resonance imaging tractography using a bootstrap approach. Magn. Reson. Med. **53**(5), 1143–1149 (2005)
14. Bayer, J., Blake, R., Plank, G., Trayanova, N.: A novel rule-based algorithm for assigning myocardial fiber orientation to computational heart models. Ann. Biomed. Eng. **40**(10), 2243–2254 (2012)
15. Nagler, A., Bertoglio, C., Stoeck, C.T., Kozerske, S., Wall, W.A.: Cardiac fibres estimation from arbitrarily spaced difusion tensor MRI. In: Lecture Notes in Computer Science. vol. 9126, pp. 198–206. Springer, Heidelberg (2015)
16. Hsu, E., Muzikant, A., Matulevicius, S., Penland, R., Henriquez, C.: Magnetic resonance myocardial fiber-orientation mapping with direct histological correlation. Am. J. Physiol. Heart Circulatory Physiol. **274**(5), H1627–H1634 (1998)
17. Scollan, D.F., Holmes, A., Winslow, R., Forder, J.: Histological validation of myocardial microstructure obtained from diffusion tensor magnetic resonance imaging. Am. J. Physiol. Heart Circulatory Physiol. **275**(6), H2308–H2318 (1998)
18. Freytag, B., Wang, V.Y., Christie, G.R., Wilson, A.J., Sands, G.B., LeGrice, I.J., Young, A.A., Nash, M.P.: Field-based parameterisation of cardiac muscle structure from diffusion tensors. FIMH 2015. LNCS, vol. 9126, pp. 146–154. Springer, Heidelberg (2015)
19. LeGrice, I.J., Hunter, P.J., Smaill, B.: Laminar structure of the heart: a mathematical model. Am. J. Physiol. Heart Circulatory Physiol. **272**, H2466–H2476 (1997)
20. Christie, G., Bullivant, D., Blackett, S., Hunter, P.J.: Modelling and visualising the heart. Comput. Vis. Sci. **4**(4), 227–235 (2002)
21. Basser, P.J., Pierpaoli, C.: Microstructural and physiological features of tissues elucidated by quantitative-diffusion-tensor MRI. J. Mag. Reson. Series B **111**, 209–219 (1996)

Confidence Measures for Assessing the HARP Algorithm in Tagged Magnetic Resonance Imaging

Hanne Kause[1]([⊠]), Aura Hernàndez-Sabaté[4], Patricia Márquez-Valle[4], Andrea Fuster[2,3], Luc Florack[2,3], Hans van Assen[1], and Debora Gil[4]

[1] Department of Electrical Engineering, Eindhoven University of Technology, Eindhoven, The Netherlands
h.b.kause@tue.nl
[2] Department of Biomedical Engineering, Eindhoven University of Technology, Eindhoven, The Netherlands
[3] Department of Mathematics and Computer Science, Eindhoven University of Technology, Eindhoven, The Netherlands
[4] Computer Vision Center and Computer Science Department, Universitat Autònoma de Barcelona, Bellaterra, Barcelona, Spain

Abstract. Cardiac deformation and changes therein have been linked to pathologies. Both can be extracted in detail from tagged Magnetic Resonance Imaging (tMRI) using harmonic phase (HARP) images. Although point tracking algorithms have shown to have high accuracies on HARP images, these vary with position. Detecting and discarding areas with unreliable results is crucial for use in clinical support systems. This paper assesses the capability of two confidence measures (CMs), based on energy and image structure, for detecting locations with reduced accuracy in motion tracking results. These CMs were tested on a database of simulated tMRI images containing the most common artifacts that may affect tracking accuracy. CM performance is assessed based on its capability for HARP tracking error bounding and compared in terms of significant differences detected using a multi comparison analysis of variance that takes into account the most influential factors on HARP tracking performance. Results showed that the CM based on image structure was better suited to detect unreliable optical flow vectors. In addition, it was shown that CMs can be used to detect optical flow vectors with large errors in order to improve the optical flow obtained with the HARP tracking algorithm.

1 Introduction

Tagged MRI (tMRI) is an important imaging technique to obtain detailed motion information of the cardiac left ventricle (LV) [1]. Tagged MRI images are obtained by spatially modulating the MR magnetization (SPAMM) field just before performing a cine acquisition so that images have a characteristic stripe or grid pattern that deforms along with cardiac tissue contraction and relaxation [2]. This enables the analysis of motion and deformation over time, which

© Springer International Publishing Switzerland 2016
O. Camara et al. (Eds.): STACOM 2015, LNCS 9534, pp. 69–79, 2016.
DOI: 10.1007/978-3-319-28712-6_8

are known to reflect changes due to pathology [3–5]. The current standard for obtaining motion information from tMRI is by application of a material point tracking algorithm on harmonic phase (HARP) images, presented by Osman et al. [6,7]. In the past, it has been shown that HARP tracking is able to correctly estimate the displacement of the cardiac muscle [8,9]. Nevertheless, there will always be a limit to the accuracy which may drop in difficult areas. Therefore, it is important to provide an estimate of the upper bound for the error by means of a confidence measure (CM).

In this paper, we test the suitability of two CMs to serve as an estimation of the error bounds in the absence of ground truth. The proposed CMs are quantities computed from the input data that should help detect those points for which the tracking is not accurate enough for further use, such as strain computations. Unreliable points can be selected for post-processing by CMs, which improves the quality of the results. It should be noted that for each value of the confidence measure, which in our case lies within $[0, 1]$, it can only provide an upper bound to the displacement error at each pixel, instead of the displacement error value itself (according to numerical error analysis [10]). This implies that high values of the confidence measure, i.e. high confidence, should ensure a low tracking error, while for low CM values errors may take any value, even a small one. Points that have a high value of the CM and a high error are unpredictable points, which cannot be detected by the CM and, thus, should not occur if the confidence measure has a perfect performance. Furthermore, when this behaviour is stable across frames or references with similar features, the CM is suited for bounding the error in the absence of ground truth, which is ultimately what we need to apply the CMs in a clinical setting.

To the best knowledge of the authors, no confidence measures have been proposed that can give an estimate of the upper bound of the displacement error in HARP results. In this paper, we propose and test the capability of different CMs for bounding the motion estimation error of the HARP algorithm, which is explained in Sect. 3, while tracking the cardiac left ventricle in tMRI sequences. First, a database of synthetic tagged MR images containing several motion patterns with known ground truth was generated by means of a simplified cardiac motion simulator [11,12] and is analysed with the HARP tracking algorithm. Second, sparse-density plots [13] were used to quantify the capability of a given CM to bound the displacement error within the myocardium. Statistical analysis over the variability of sparse-density plots is used to test the impact of motion and appearance factors in displacement accuracy.

2 Evaluation of Confidence Measures

In this work, the goal of a confidence measure is to provide an upper bound for the flow error in order to detect pixels for which the flow estimation is likely to be non-reliable. In order to assess the capability of a CM for bounding the displacement error, we use Sparse-Density Plots (SDPs) [13]. An SDP evaluates the risk of a confidence measure; that is, the proportion of points (ρ) the bound of which can not be determined by CM values. While decision support systems usually set a lower bound to acceptable accuracy, we compute ρ in terms of the maximum allowed error (E_{max}), which we call risk:

$$\rho(CM_0) := P(E > E_{max}|CM > CM_0). \tag{1}$$

Consequently the SDP is the plot given by:

$$SDP(prct_{CM}) := (prct_{CM}, \rho(prct_{CM})), \tag{2}$$

where $prct_{CM}$ are CM distribution percentiles , which are used instead of directly using the CM to ensure that the SDP is invariant under monotonically increasing transformations of the CM.

Considering a database of image sequences with ground truth, we compute the SDP profile for every two subsequent frames. Note that each SDP profile assesses a bound on the optical flow error specifically for the two frames on which it was based. However, we would like to obtain a general curve, $\mathcal{SDP}$, that can reliably assess a bound on the optical flow error (also called risk) for any other sequence with similar features without ground truth. Therefore, we provide a statistical bound for the risk by computing an upper estimator of SDP profiles using a Student's t-distribution for confident estimation of random variables means. Let us consider a sample of SDP profiles, $\{SDP_i\}_{i=1}^N$ of N frames ($N > 30$) presenting similar motion and appearance features. For each CM percentile, $prct_{CM}$, consider the sample mean, $\mu(prct_{CM})$, and variance, $\sigma(prct_{CM})$, computed for the values $\rho_i(prct_{CM})$, $i = 1, \ldots, N$. Then, an upper bound for $\rho_i(prct_{CM})$ at confidence level $\alpha_{\mathcal{SDP}}$ is given by:

$$\mu(prct_{CM}) + t_{1-\alpha_{\mathcal{SDP}}}^{N-1}\sigma(prct_{CM}) = \Upsilon_{prct_{CM}} \tag{3}$$

for $t_{1-\alpha_{\mathcal{SDP}}}^{N-1}$ the value of a Student's t-distribution with N-1 degrees of freedom having a cumulative probability equal to $1 - \alpha_{\mathcal{SDP}}$ [14]. The bounding curve is defined as

$$\mathcal{SDP} := \mathcal{SDP}(prct_{CM}) = (prct_{CM}, \Upsilon_{prct_{CM}})$$

and it indicates that, once a $prct_{CM}$ of pixels has been removed, the error of the remaining ones should be under EE_{max} with probability $\Upsilon_{prct_{CM}}$.

By definition of the confidence interval, the risk at $prct_{CM}$ is under $\Upsilon_{prct_{CM}}$ for new incoming frames with probability $1 - \alpha_{\mathcal{SDP}}$ [14], that is, for approximately $(1 - \alpha_{\mathcal{SDP}})\%$ of frames. For the remaining $\alpha_{\mathcal{SDP}}\%$, the risk could be as high as 1. The bound $\Upsilon_{prct_{CM}}$ applies to all frames provided that SDP variability across such a frame sample is not large [15]. In this context, a most relevant quality feature of confidence measures is a stable behaviour of SDP across sequences in the decision support system. In other words, the lower variability in training SDP profiles we have, the higher predictive value $\mathcal{SDP}$ has.

Under the previous considerations, the capability of a CM for risk bounding should follow a two-stage cascade process. First, $\mathcal{SDP}$ predictive value should be assessed and, then, for those CMs with the highest predictive value, the quality of the bound provided by $\mathcal{SDP}$ should be determined. The predictive value is assessed by the variance of $\mathcal{SDP}$ across the training samples, while the quality of $\mathcal{SDP}$ bound is measured in terms of a minimum risk for the bounded pixels. Each quality score is defined as follows:

1. $\mathcal{SDP}$ **Predictive Value.** Given a sampling of CM-percentiles $prct_{CM}^j = \frac{j \cdot h}{N_{prct}}$, with h the sampling step and N_{prct} the number of percentiles, the variance of its $\mathcal{SDP}$ is approximated by the unbiased sample estimator:

$$\sigma_i^{\mathcal{SDP}} = \frac{1}{N_{prct} - 1} \sum_{j=1}^{N_{prct}} \left(\rho_i(prct_{CM}^j) - \Upsilon_{prct_{CM}}^j \right)^2, \tag{4}$$

where i and j correspond to the frame and the percentile, respectively, and $\Upsilon_{prct_{CM}}^j$ is the sample mean at the j-th sampled percentile computed by (3).

2. $\mathcal{SDP}$ **Bound Quality.** The amount of risk for a family of SDP curves can be summarized by the mean area, AUC_i^{SDP}, under the curve SDP_i. Given a sampling of CM-percentiles $prct_{CM}^j = \frac{j \cdot h}{N_{prct}}$, AUC_i^{SDP} is defined as:

$$AUC_i^{SDP} := \frac{1}{N_{prct}} \sum_{j=1}^{N_{prct}} \rho_i(prct_{CM}^j) \tag{5}$$

for i, j denoting the frame and CM-percentile, respectively.

Figure 1 illustrates the computation of the two quality scores, the variance $\sigma_i^{\mathcal{SDP}}$ and the average risk AUC_i^{SDP}. The prediction curve $\mathcal{SDP}$ is plotted in black and the SDP_i in red. Subsequently, the variance $\sigma_i^{\mathcal{SDP}}$ is given by the area between both curves (shaded area in Fig. 1(a)) whereas the risk AUC_i^{SDP} is given by the area under the curve (shaded area in Fig. 1(b)).

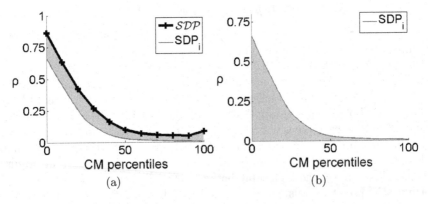

Fig. 1. CM quality assessment: $\sigma_i^{\mathcal{SDP}}$ computation for $\mathcal{SDP}$ predictive value assessment (a), and AUC_i^{SDP} computation for $\mathcal{SDP}$ bound quality (b).

3 The HARP Algorithm

The stripe or grid pattern that is present in tMRI images deforms along with myocardial tissue contraction and relaxation. This means that via feature tracking, assessment of local cardiac motion should be possible. Osman et al. developed a tracking algorithm (HARP) [6] that links changes of the feature *over time* to local *spatial* feature changes by the tissue displacement $y^{(n+1)} - y^{(n)}$ to be estimated, similar to optical flow [16], but now iteratively:

$$\underbrace{\mathbf{y}^{(n+1)} - \mathbf{y}^{(n)}}_{\text{displacement}} = -\underbrace{\left[\nabla^*\mathbf{a}(\mathbf{y}^{(n)}, t_{m+1})\right]^{-1}}_{\text{(spatial) feature gradient}} \underbrace{\mathcal{W}(\mathbf{a}(\mathbf{y}^{(n)}, t_{m+1}) - \mathbf{a}(\mathbf{y}_m, t_m))}_{\text{temporal feature derivative}}. \quad (6)$$

Here, $\mathbf{y}$ is two-dimensional position, n is the iteration number, t_m is time, $\mathbf{a}$ is the *apparent* feature vector $[a_1\ a_2]$, where the subscript determines the input image (image 1 and 2 start with perpendicular stripe tags in the first frame), and $\mathcal{W}$ indicates the apparent feature is wrapped (v.i.).

Typically, the feature tracking in both optical flow and HARP assume feature constancy over time. However, since the intensity of material points is not constant in tMRI images, due to signal decay as a result of T_1-relaxation, intensity is not a proper feature to track. To overcome this issue, Osman et al. developed a tracking algorithm based on (instead of pixel intensity) the harmonic phase of material points, unaffected by signal decay [6].

By application of a Gabor filter to isolate the i-th spectral peak at frequency ω_i in the Fourier domain, a complex-valued spatial domain image is obtained. Usually, the first harmonic spectral peak in the tag direction is preserved. Then, the harmonic phase image is obtained by taking the argument of each pixel in the complex spatial domain image. This is in fact not the true phase ϕ_k but the wrapped "apparent" phase a_k which lies within the interval $[-\pi, \pi)$.

Because $\mathbf{a}$ is wrapped, it has discontinuities, which leads to problems in the context of computing gradients. Therefore, before computing $\nabla \mathbf{a}$, $\mathbf{a}$ is locally unwrapped, indicated by ∇^* in Eq. (6).

4 Experimental Settings

The goal of our experiments is to show the applicability of the framework for selecting CMs capable of predicting the displacement error upper bound in cardiac tagged MRI sequences analysed with HARP. Since the commercially available HARP software does not allow access to the calculations, we used an in-house implementation of the HARP algorithm described by Osman et al. [6]. In the experiments, we are interested in the displacement of each pixel in the myocardium at each time step and, therefore, we apply the HARP algorithm at each frame separately. In [6], iteration stops when the phase difference between source and target position drops below a threshold. However, since phase error is part of our CM, we did not want to use it as a stopping criterion. Consequently, a stopping criterion based on phase error stability ($\Delta\phi < 0.01$) and/or maximum number of iterations (N = 30) was implemented.

The iteration process is stopped when the last five estimates are stable with a threshold of 0.01 or when the maximum number of 30 iterations is reached.

To find the optimal confidence measure for the HARP tracking algorithm, we have considered two types of CMs:

1. Image structure (C_k). The condition numbers of the spatial harmonic phase gradient matrix from each iteration, see Eq. (6), defined as

$$C_k = s_{min}/s_{max}$$

where s are singular values [17], are combined by taking the L^2-norm.

2. Energy (C_e). The confidence measure $C_e = \cos(\phi)$ is computed from the final temporal harmonic phase difference

$$\phi = \mathcal{W}(\mathbf{a}(\mathbf{y}_{m+1}, t_{m+1}) - \mathbf{a}(\mathbf{y}_m, t_m)),$$

which is the difference between the harmonic phases a of the material point in the two frames, with $\mathcal{W}$ a wrapping function, see Eq. (6).

4.1   Cardiac Deformation DataSet

In order to test if CMs can accurately bound the motion tracking error, it is necessary to have images with a known motion field. A solution for this is to use artificially generated images. However, to reliably apply the CMs to real

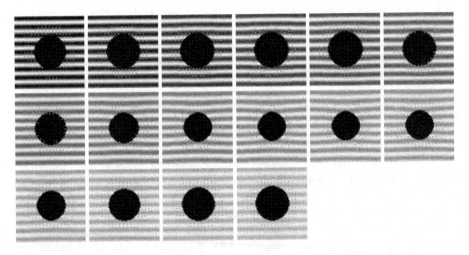

Fig. 2. Frames of horizontal tagging sequence from the 3rd slice of the set with contraction. The arrows illustrate a sample of the ground truth and are amplified three times for visibility.

data, these synthetic images need to have comparable features to the real clinical images. Therefore, we use the database of synthetic MR images (Fig. 2) first introduced by Márquez-Valle et al. [12], which is based on the cardiac motion simulator by Arts et al. incorporating a time-dependent model using 13 parameters [18].

The datasets contain simulated sinusoidal SPAMM tagged sequences [2], which are modelled with signal decay according to [11]. Different image datasets were created containing either rotation around the long-axis or radially-dependent contraction, while eliminating longitudinal motion in the model to prevent out-of-plane motion in the short-axis images. All seven short-axis slices existed of 50×50 isotropic pixels and started with the longitudinal axis in the center of the image, see Fig. 2. The cardiac cycle was split into 16 frames and the tagged period was set to 6.6 pixels in either horizontal or vertical direction. Rician noise was added with an SNR of 25, which was constant over time. SNR was defined as SNR $= \frac{\mu}{\sigma}$ with μ the mean signal and σ the standard deviation of the noise [19]. Signal decay is modelled to mimic the T_1 decay present in MRI. For details on the synthetic data generation, see [12].

4.2   Statistical Analysis

Significance in $\mathcal{SDP}$ variability and bound quality is checked using ANOVA, which is a powerful statistical tool for detecting differences in performance across methodologies as well as the impact of different factors or assumptions. We can apply ANOVA in case our data consists of one or several categorical explanatory variables (called factors) and a quantitative response of the variable. The variability analysis is defined after the ANOVA quantitative score and the different factors and methods are determined. Training data (individuals) is grouped according to such factors, and differences among quantitative response group means are computed. ANOVA provides a statistical way to assess if such differences are significant enough for a given confidence level α. In case of having more than one factor, ANOVA also detects any interaction across the different factors that might distort the analysis of results for each factor separately. If interaction across factors is significant, then the multiple ANOVA has to be re-designed as one factor ANOVA combining all factor groups into a single one to determine whether or not the response variable depends on the combined factors.

The ANOVA design (variable, individuals and factors) for each quality score ($\mathcal{SDP}$ Predictive Value and $\mathcal{SDP}$ Bound Quality) is defined taking as factors the confidence measures (with groups defined by C_e, C_k) and cardiac motions (with groups defined by Contraction, Rotation). The sampling for each CM quality score is given by $\{\sigma_i^{\mathcal{SDP}}\}_{i=1}^{N_{Fr}}$ and $\{AUC_i^{\mathcal{SDP}}\}_{i=1}^{N_{Fr}}$, respectively. In these experiments the number of frames, N_{Fr}, is set to 40 and they have been randomly sampled across the SA sequences with rotation and contraction motion. To account for non normality in data, ANOVA is performed in logarithmic scale.

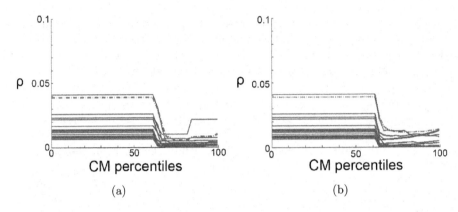

Fig. 3. SDP plots of the confidence measures C_k (a) and C_e (b) from 40 frames randomly sampled across the sequence with contracting motion.

5   Results and Discussion

Figure 3 shows the SDP plots of both confidence measures for the sequence with contracting motion. Table 1 shows the average variability (first two columns) and risk (second two columns) for each ANOVA factor group (confidence measures in columns and cardiac motions in rows). For the two quality measures, the 2-way ANOVA over CM and cardiac motions does not detect any significant differences for the motion factor (with $p - Mot = 0.18$ for σ_i^{SDP} and $p - Mot = 0.84$ for AUC_i^{SDP}) nor interaction (with $p - inter = 0.78$ for σ_i^{SDP} and $p - inter = 0.68$ for AUC_i^{SDP}). This implies that the capabilities of each CM for error bounding are independent of the cardiac motion. Conversely, the 2-way ANOVA is significant (with $p - CM = 5 \times 10^{-3}$ for σ_i^{SDP} and $p - CM = 0.005$ for AUC_i^{SDP}) in the column factor and, thus, the capability of C_e and C_k for error bounding is different. In particular, and according to the average values reported in Table 1, we conclude that C_k has a lower variability and risk, regardless of the motion ($p - inter > 0.68$). This is due to the fact that in uniform areas of the image such as the center, interpolation errors are low but HARP cannot compute the phase properly which results in bad correlation.

This is confirmed by a multi comparison test with Tukey correction for one factor given by the two CMs and variable sampling taken for the two motions. The plots of Fig. 4 show the result of the test for SDP Predictive Value

Table 1. Average variability and risk for each ANOVA factor group.

	σ_i^{SDP}		AUC_i^{SDP}	
	C_e	C_k	C_e	C_k
Contraction	2.5×10^{-3}	0.6×10^{-3}	5×10^{-3}	2×10^{-3}
Rotation	7.2×10^{-3}	0.56×10^{-3}	7.3×10^{-3}	2.7×10^{-3}

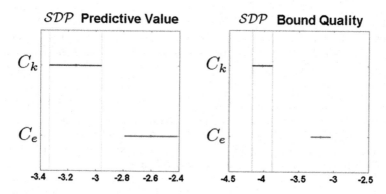

Fig. 4. Multicomparison test for $\mathcal{SDP}$ Predictive Value and $\mathcal{SDP}$ Bound Quality. Results are in logarithmic scale to account for non normality in the data.

(on the left) and $\mathcal{SDP}$ Bound Quality (on the right). Both plots show intervals for mean differences. Each level mean is represented as a horizontal line centred at the mean group and vertically distributed according to the confidence measure. In the case that there are differences between a selected interval and the others (one in this case), the non-selected intervals are depicted in red.

Note that it is not possible to give a direct and absolute upper bound of the optic flow error. However, since the presented framework uses powerful statistical tools, we are able to provide the risk of unbounded pixels for a specific confidence measure and a sequence with no ground truth. This will enable more reliable interpretation of HARP tracking results. As a next step, pixels with a low confidence could be discarded from the computation and interpolated in the final results. Another option is to include regularisation on the HARP images in the areas with low confidence.

Because the synthetic images used in this study accurately simulate the features of real tMRI sequences, we expect that our results translate to real tMRI sequences fairly well. In the future we will apply this framework to clinical images, for which (part of the) optic flow is known[1], in order to prove that these CMs indeed bound the error in clinical images as well.

6   Conclusion

In this paper, we propose and test the capability of two confidence measures for bounding several motion estimation errors of the HARP algorithm in tracking the cardiac left ventricle in tMRI sequences. A 2-way ANOVA over CMs and cardiac motions did not detect any significant differences for the motion factor nor interaction, so that the capabilities of each CM for error bounding are independent of the type of cardiac motion. Furthermore, we concluded that the

---

[1] A set of volunteer sequences and phantom images are available from the 2011 STA-COM challenge. For these images a set of feature points is tracked over time.

capability of the CM computed from image structure, C_k, has a better error bounding capability than the CM determined by the energy, C_e. In particular, the phase is not computed properly in noisy areas, which means it cannot correlate well to interpolation error.

Acknowledgements. Work supported by Spanish project TIN2012-33116. First author is supported by the Dutch Technology Foundation STW, which is part of the Netherlands Organisation for Scientic Research (NWO), and which is partly funded by the Ministry of Economic Affairs. Third author is supported by the FPI-MICINN BES-2010-031102 program. Last author is a Serra Hunter fellow.

References

1. Zerhouni, E.A., Parish, D.M., Rogers, W.J., Yang, A., Shapiro, E.P.: Human heart: tagging with MR imaging–a method for noninvasive assessment of myocardial motion. Radiology **169**(1), 59–63 (1988)
2. Axel, L., Dougherty, L.: MR imaging of motion with spatial modulation of magnetization. Radiology **171**(3), 841–845 (1989)
3. Mirsky, I., Pfeffer, J.M., Pfeffer, M.A., Braunwald, E.: The contractile state as the major determinant in the evolution of left ventricular dysfunction in the spontaneously hypertensive rat. Circ. Res. **53**, 767–778 (1983)
4. Götte, M.J., van Rossum, A.C., Twisk, J.W.R., Kuijer, J.P.A., Marcus, J.M., Visser, C.A.: Quantification of regional contractile function after infarction: strain analysis superior to wall thickening analysis in discriminating infarct from remote myocardium. J. Am. Coll. Cardiol. **37**, 808–817 (2001)
5. Delhaas, T., Kotte, J., van der Toorn, A., Snoep, G., Prinzen, F.W., Arts, T.: Increase in left ventricular torsion-to-shortening ratio in children with valvular aorta stenosis. Magn. Reson. Med. **51**, 135–139 (2004)
6. Osman, N.F., Kerwin, W.S., McVeigh, E.R., Prince, J.L.: Cardiac motion tracking using CINE harmonic phase (HARP) magnetic resonance imaging. Mag. Reson. Med. **42**(6), 1048–1060 (1999)
7. Osman, N.F., McVeigh, E.R., Prince, J.L.: Imaging heart motion using harmonic phase MRI. IEEE Trans. Med. Imaging **19**(3), 186–202 (2000)
8. Sampath, S., Derbyshire, J.A., Atalar, E., Osman, N.F., Prince, J.L.: Real-time imaging of two-dimensional cardiac strain using a harmonic phase magnetic resonance imaging (HARP-MRI) pulse sequence. Mag. Reson. Med. **50**(1), 154–163 (2003)
9. Kraitchman, D.L., Sampath, S., Castillo, E., Derbyshire, J.A., Boston, R.C., Bluemke, D.A., Gerber, B.L., Prince, J.L., Osman, N.F.: Quantitative ischemia detection during cardiac magnetic resonance stress testing by use of fastharp. Circulation **107**, 2025–2030 (2003)
10. Cheney, W., Kincaid, D.: Numerical Mathematics and Computing, 6th edn. Bob Pirtle, USA (2008)
11. Waks, E., Prince, J.L., Douglas, A.S.: Cardiac motion simulator for tagged MRI. In: Workshop on Mathematical Methods in Biomedical Image Analysis (MMBIA 1996) (1996). 0182

12. Márquez-Valle, P., Kause, H., Fuster, A., Hernández-Sabaté, A., Florack, L., Gil, D., van Assen, H.C.: Factors affecting optical flow performance in tagging magnetic resonance imaging. In: Camara, O., Mansi, T., Pop, M., Rhode, K., Sermesant, M., Young, A. (eds.) STACOM 2014. LNCS, vol. 8896, pp. 231–238. Springer, Heidelberg (2015)

13. Márquez-Valle, P., Gil, D., Hernàndez-Sabaté, A.: Evaluation of the capabilities of confidence measures for assessing optical flow quality. In: International Conference on Computer Vision - Workshops (2013)

14. Fisher, R.: Statistical Methods and Scientific Inference. Oliver and Boyd, Edinburgh (1956)

15. Newbold, P., Carlson, W., Thorne, B.: Statistics for Business and Economics. Pearson Education, New York (2007)

16. Van Assen, H., Florack, L., Simonis, F., Westenberg, J., Strijkers, G.: Cardiac strain and rotation analysis using multi-scale optical flow. In: Wittek, A., Nielsen, P.M.F., Miller, K. (eds.) Computational Biomechanics for Medicine V, pp. 89–100. Springer, Heidelberg (2010)

17. Márquez-Valle, P., Gil, D., Hernàndez-Sabaté, A.: A complete confidence framework for optical flow. In: Fusiello, A., Murino, V., Cucchiara, R. (eds.) ECCV 2012 Ws/Demos, Part II. LNCS, vol. 7584, pp. 124–133. Springer, Heidelberg (2012)

18. Arts, T., Hunter, W., Douglas, A., Muijtjens, A., Reneman, R.: Description of the deformation of the left ventricle by a kinematic model. J. Biomech. $25(10)$, 1119–1127 (1992)

19. Gutberlet, M., Schwinge, K., Freyhardt, P., et al.: Influence of high magnetic field strengths and parallel acquisition strategies on image quality in cardiac 2D CINE magnetic resonance imaging. Eur. Radiol. $15(8)$, 1586–1597 (2005)

Papillary Muscle Segmentation from a Multi-atlas Database: A Feasibility Study

Benedetta Biffi[1,2]($\boxtimes$), Maria A. Zuluaga[3], Sébastien Ourselin[3],
Andrew M. Taylor[2,4], and Silvia Schievano[2,4]

[1] UCL Department of Medical Physics and Biomedical Engineering,
University College London, London, UK
b.biffi@ucl.ac.uk
[2] Great Ormond Street Hospital for Children, London, UK
[3] Translational Imaging Group, Centre for Medical Image Computing,
University College London, London, UK
[4] UCL Institute of Cardiovascular Science, University College London, London, UK

Abstract. Planning of mitral valve replacement would benefit from pre-procedural 3D models that could allow the clinician to fully understand the patient anatomical and functional condition. However, no single image modality can provide the complete picture alone but 3D echocardiography and magnetic resonance imaging (MRI) could be combined to leverage the advantages of each modality. The fusion of cardiac echo and MR images is a challenging task that currently requires the use of anatomical landmarks to drive the registration. In mitral valve treatment planning, the papillary muscles represent an ideal landmark set as they can be clearly identified in both image modalities. In this paper, we address the problem of papillary muscles automatic segmentation from MRI by proposing an atlas-based segmentation method. Results show that a good quality segmentation (Dice score 0.60 ± 0.14 and 0.73 ± 0.06 for anterior and posterior papillary muscle, respectively) can be achieved within the straightforward pipeline provided by this approach, also on images acquired with different scanners. Hence, our atlas-based segmentation method could represent the first key step towards a novel, automated echo and MRI fusion algorithm.

1 Introduction

Mitral valve (MV) regurgitation is a common form of valvular abnormality which requires treatment or replacement through invasive open-heart surgery, with considerable risks of significant morbidity and mortality [1]. Thus, there is an increased demand for minimally invasive techniques, such as sutureless and/or transcatheter MV replacement. These procedures have already been developed and successfully used for the replacement of aortic and pulmonary valves, and only recently techniques are becoming available for the MV, as its anatomy is complex, with a non-uniform geometry that relies on several inter-related components for its function: the annulus, the leaflets, the chordae tendineae, and the supporting papillary muscles. Echocardiography is the conventional

© Springer International Publishing Switzerland 2016
O. Camara et al. (Eds.): STACOM 2015, LNCS 9534, pp. 80–89, 2016.
DOI: 10.1007/978-3-319-28712-6_9

image modality for MV assessment, offering real-time structural and functional information. With the latest advances in ultrasound probes, high-resolution, full-volume imaging and quantification of the morphology of the entire MV apparatus have become feasible. Magnetic resonance imaging (MRI) is the reference standard for the measurement of ventricular and atrial size, geometry and function. By combining these two imaging modalities, it would be possible to fill in information missing from echocardiography or MRI alone to create a detailed 3D model of the left heart and MV.

A pre-requisite for the creation of a fused model is the alignment of both image modalities. This is a big challenge as the 3D registration of echocardiography to MRI remains an open problem. To date, most approaches for echo-to-MRI (or computed tomography, CT) registration have been developed for neurosurgical applications [2,3]. Cardiac echo-to-MRI registration has been limitedly addressed [4–6]. Currently developed methods require either some manual initial registration [4,5] or the definition of landmarks [6] in both images that can guide the registration procedure. Landmark-based approaches [6] for echo-to-MRI registration represent a good trade-off between accuracy, ease of use and computational time. However, for heart images there are only few spatially accurate anatomical landmarks. Moreover, due to the limited field of view (FOV) of echocardiography, it is mandatory to define landmarks that are specific to the problem (*i.e.* anatomical region) addressed.

Within the context of mitral valve treatment planning, the papillary muscles (PMs) represent an ideal landmark set as they can be clearly identified in both echo and MRI images (Fig. 1), and their successfull adoption has been previously documented. Savi et al. [7] rigidly registered cardiac PET and echo images by using PMs and the inferior junction of the right ventricle as reference points. PMs were used as landmarks also in [8] to validate a rigid, surface-based, cardiac

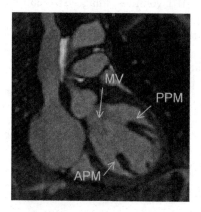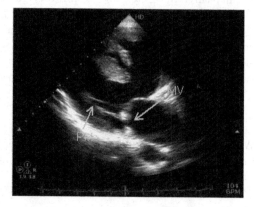

Fig. 1. Papillary muscles highlighted in both image modalities. (a) Coronal view of cardiac whole-heart MRI. The papillary muscles are highlighted by the red arrows. Details of the chordae and the MV leaflets are also visible. (b) Parasternal long-axis view of 3D echo (Color figure online).

MR-PET registration. With the final aim of fusing 3D echo and MRI for MV pre-procedural planning, in this work we first address the problem of accurately extracting the PMs from MR images.

While the segmentation of the main chambers of the heart has been widely addressed [9], little work has focused on the extraction of smaller structures such as the PMs. Spreeuwers et al. [10] were the first to tackle the problem through a 2D region-based approach. More recently, Gao et al. [11] addressed the problem through a topological method that tries to restore missing structures from an initial segmentation using high resolution CT. Other methods in the literature have extracted the PMs along with the left ventricle but, not as a separate structure. Despite the popularity of atlas-based methods in the segmentation of the heart [9,12], none of the existing work has tried to use this type of framework for the segmentation of the PMs. This could be explained by the complexity, shape, size and position variability of this structure. The final aim of this work is to demonstrate, through a validation study, that atlas-based approaches are well suited for PMs segmentation.

The remaining of this paper is organised as follows: Sect. 2 describes the data and the specific methods used in this study. Section 3 shows the results. Finally, a discussion on the obtained results and a conclusion are presented in Sect. 4.

2   Materials and Methods

In this section we describe the data, the motivation for an atlas-based approach and the evaluation scheme used to assess PMs segmentation.

2.1   Materials

Twenty-three 3D ECG- and respiratory-gated MRI volumes, images size $256 \times 256 \times 140$, were acquired at King's College London [13]. We denote this as set S_1. Two additional 3D Whole Heart ECG- and respiratory-gated MRI datasets, image size $152 \times 256 \times 120$ and $128 \times 256 \times 96$, were acquired at Great Ormond Street Hospital, London, using a different scanner (1.5 Tesla Siemens Avanto). We denote this as set S_2. Both datasets come from healthy volunteers.

2.2   Method

We make use of a multi-atlas based segmentation approach. In the following, we describe the atlas creation, the selected atlas segmentation method and the evaluation scheme.

Atlas Creation. For each scan from S_1, a manual segmentation of the four main chambers, the myocardium, the pulmonary artery and the aorta was available. ITK-SNAP [14] was adopted to add the labels of the antero-lateral (APM) and postero-medial (PPM) papillary muscles (Fig. 2). To ease the labelling task, an initial segmentation was obtained with the Snake toolbox. The region of interest was selected around each muscle and a thresholding filter applied to correctly drive the active contour evolution. One or more balloons were placed within each muscle main region and the snake evolution performed until convergence imposing expanding balloon force and low curvature constraint. Manual editing was performed in the obtained result to correct for errors caused by the irregular and branched shape of the PMs.

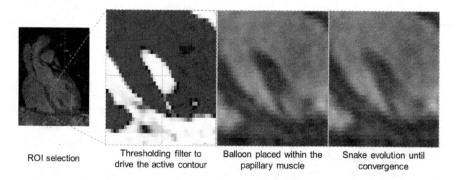

| ROI selection | Thresholding filter to drive the active contour | Balloon placed within the papillary muscle | Snake evolution until convergence |

Fig. 2. Semi-automated segmentation method adopted to label the PMs. ITK-SNAP [14] was adopted for this purpose.

Using the available labels for S_1, two different atlases were created. An atlas set containing all the possible available labels (whole heart and PMs), which we denoted as $WHPMA$, and an atlas set containing only the labels of the PMs. We denoted this atlas as set PMA. Set S_2 was not included in the atlas and was only used for validation purposes.

Multi-atlas Segmentation. There is a wide range of multi-atlas based approaches addressing the problem of cardiac segmentation [9]. We have selected to use the segmentation pipeline proposed by Zuluaga et al. [12] as it has shown to be robust in the segmentation of different structures within the heart [15,16]. The details of the presented method can be found in [12]. Here we only give a brief description of it.

Let an atlas database A be expressed as the set of n paired images $A = \{Y_j; L_j\}$, $j \in \{1, ..., n\}$, with Y_j an intensity image and L_j a label image, and let Y_u be an unseen image to be diagnosed. A segmentation for Y_u is obtained by transforming the set of n atlases into the image space of Y_u and then applying a fusion criterion to combine the label images L_j from each atlas into a consensus segmentation $\hat{L}_u$. To determine whether an unseen image Y_u contains a specific pathology, it has to be segmented using an atlas set with the same pathological pattern.

The structures surrounding the heart tend to bias the registration in cardiac images. To avoid this problem, the atlas set A is registered to Y_u in a two-stage process. In the first stage, a region of interest that encloses the heart is obtained by affinely registering Y_u to every Y_j, applying the obtained transformations to binarised L_j images, and finally fusing those into a mask M_u using a majority voting criterion. In the second stage, this mask is applied to the unseen image to allow for flexible registrations without bias. With a nonrigid free form deformation registration using normalised mutual information, we align the entire atlas set A to Y_u.

The final segmentation $\hat{L}_u$ is obtained by using the multi-STEPS algorithm [17] in combination with a locally normalised cross correlation (LNCC) based ranking strategy to determine which are the most suitable atlases to use in the fusion process. The STEPS algorithm provides a parameter X that allows the control of the number of atlases to be used locally according to the LNCC.

Evaluation Scheme. The capability of the multi-atlas segmentation method to obtain a satisfactory extraction of the PMs was evaluated using a leave-one-out cross validation scheme on set S_1, *i.e.* each image was automatically segmented adopting the remaining twenty-two as atlas. Two different tests were performed, the first using $WHPMA$, and the second using PMA.

The obtained results were compared with the manual segmentation in terms of visual assessment and Dice score, the latter computed as

$$Dice = \frac{2(V_{manual} \cap V_{automatic})}{(V_{manual} \cup V_{automatic})} \tag{1}$$

Additionally, the PMs from S_2 were segmented with $WHPMA$ using the complete set (23 images). Visual assessment and Dice scores were computed also for this dataset. The goal of this experiment was to determine the sensibility of the method to different image scanners.

3   Validation and Results

Cross-Validation. The proposed method succeeded in performing the segmentation of all the twenty-three volumes of S_1, when both $WHPMA$ and PMA were adopted.

Table 1 shows the results of computing the Dice scores for both the APM and PPM segmentations in S_1. The values were averaged between the twenty-three datasets and the standard deviation was computed. A reduction of the mean Dice scores is noticeable when the atlas adopted (PMA) had only the PMs labels.

In Fig. 3, the manual segmentation of one image of S_1 is compared against the one obtained with the multi-atlas approach. The automatic method was able to correctly segment all the cardiac structures and the two PMs in all the tested datasets, although the regions presenting thin and irregular branches remained difficult to label. As a result of the label fusion, the great majority of the obtained segmentation showed PMs with a more homogeneous and smooth shape than

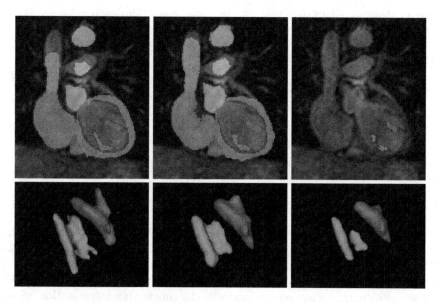

Fig. 3. Coronal views and 3D rendering of the whole heart segmentation, with particular focus on APM (green) and PPM (red). (a) Ground truth manual segmentation. (b) Automatic segmentation obtained with the fully labelled atlas. (c) Automatic segmentation obtained with the atlas where only the papillary muscles labels were provided (Color figure online).

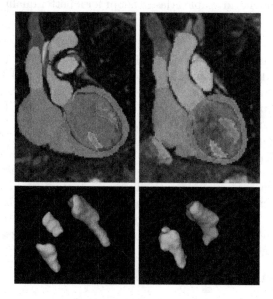

Fig. 4. Result of applying the automatic segmentation method with the proposed atlas on two new datasets acquired with different scanner and MRI sequences. Coronal view and 3D rendering of the papillary muscles segmentation.

Table 1. Mean, standard deviation (St Dev), maximum (Max) and minimum (Min) Dice scores computed between manual and multi-atlas segmentation for each image of the atlas. Results are shown when adopting the completely labelled atlas $WHPMA$ and the one with only the papillaries labels PMA.

Dice	APM		PPM	
	$WHPMA$	PMA	$WHPMA$	PMA
Mean	0.60	0.51	0.73	0.71
St Dev	0.14	0.19	0.06	0.10
Max	0.77	0.73	0.81	0.83
Min	0.22	0.00	0.62	0.41

the ground truth structures, hence influencing the values of the Dice scores. The results of adopting the atlas with only the PMs labels (PMA) are presented in Fig. 3, showing worsening of the segmentation, and suggesting the importance of the surrounding structures to guide through a correct identification of the PMs.

The average time required to perform the automatic segmentation of an unseen image, adopting atlases with twenty-two subjects, was 70 ± 5 min for whole heart ($WHPMA$) segmentation and 66 ± 1 min for only PMs segmentation (PMA). As expected, due to the reduced number of labels to compute, the segmentation with PMA results, on average, quicker than the segmentation with $WHPMA$. However, the difference in time is negligible (5 %), and $WHPMA$ remains the advisable atlas to adopt for a better quality and complete segmentation.

Application. When adopting the validated atlas $WHPMA$ from S_1 to segment two unseen datasets acquired with different machines and MRI sequences, promising results are obtained.

Dice scores computed on $S_{2,1}$ are 0.77 for APM and 0.78 for PPM, while those computed on $S_{2,2}$ are 0.69 for APM and 0.74 for PPM. With respect to the Dice scores computed in the cross-validation experiment, we observe higher Dice scores for $S_{2,1}$, while those of $S_{2,2}$ are perfectly matching the found range. This suggests that our multi-atlas segmentation method is robust in segmenting whole heart MR images acquired with different environmental conditions.

In Fig. 4 one can notice a good identification of all the cardiac structures and of the PMs, adding credit to the capability of the method in automatically identifying and precisely labelling most of the cardiac structures of interest.

4   Discussion and Conclusions

In this work we have presented the usage of a whole heart multi-atlas segmentation framework for the extraction of the PMs from MRI. Despite the popularity of atlas-based methods in cardiac imaging, no previous work had attempted the segmentation of the PMs under this framework. Although the PMs have an irregular, branched shape and their identification within the left ventricle is strictly influenced by the image quality and contrast, we have demonstrated that an atlas-based segmentation method can be adopted as a robust and feasible strategy for their identification and labelling. The algorithm performed better than a previous 2D approach using the same image modality [10].

We evaluated two different atlas sets: one containing only the PMs and another one containing labels for other structures of the heart. The results suggest that the use of extra labels enhances the quality of the segmentation. Further improvements of the segmentation could be achieved if an extra refinement step could be applied to the results, as proposed in [11]. However, the obtained quality is considered sufficient for our final aim. Furthermore, it is preferable to have one single segmentation framework rather than a complex pipeline connecting different methods.

The main challenges encountered with the developed methodology were the correct classification of the PMs with respect to the left ventricle, and the precise representation of the branched structure of the muscles. In order to improve the quality of the results, the algorithm could be extended with a further step, *i.e.* the segmentation of the PMs alone could be performed after masking the surrounding structures with a mask corresponding to the left ventricle, obtained with a preliminary full-heart segmentation. Nevertheless, we believe that the quality of the segmentation obtained within this work is sufficient for our scope, *i.e.* automatic landmark detection. In conclusion, the adoption of this method for the segmentation of the PMs in MRI is the first key step for the development of a multi-modality fusion method able to combine MRI and 3D echocardiography of the mitral valve apparatus. To the best of our knowledge, this is the first time that a fully automated segmentation method is successfully applied to MRI for the extraction of the PMs.

Acknowledgments. BB is funded by UCL EPSRC Centre for Doctoral Training in Medical Imaging Scholarship Award. SO receives funding from the EPSRC (EP/H046410/1, EP/J020990 / 1, EP/K005278), the MRC (MR/ J01107X/1), the EU-FP7 project VPH-DARE@ IT (FP7-ICT-2011-9-601055), the NIHR Biomedical Research Unit (Dementia) at UCL and the National Institute for Health Research University College London Hospitals Biomedical Research Centre (NIHR BRC UCLH/UCL High Impact Initiative). AMT and SS receive funding from Heart Research UK, the British Heart Foundation and the National Institute for Health Research Biomedical Research Centre at GOSH and UCL.

References

1. McCarthy, K.P., Ring, L., Rana, B.S.: Anatomy of the mitral valve: understanding the mitral valve complex in mitral regurgitation. Eur. Heart J. Cardiovasc. Imaging **11**(10), i3–i9 (2010)
2. Reinertsen, I., Descoteaux, M., Siddiqi, K., Collins, D.: Validation of vessel-based registration for correction of brain shift. Med. Image Anal. **11**, 374–388 (2007)

3. Rivaz, H., Chen, S.S., Collins, D.: Automatic deformable MR-ultrasound registration for image-guided neurosurgery. IEEE Trans. Med. Imaging **34**(2), 366–380 (2015)
4. Huang, X., Hill, N.A., Ren, J., Guiraudon, G.M., Boughner, D.R., Peters, T.M.: Dynamic 3D ultrasound and MR image registration of the beating heart. In: Duncan, J.S., Gerig, G. (eds.) MICCAI 2005. LNCS, vol. 3750, pp. 171–178. Springer, Heidelberg (2005)
5. Huang, X., Hill, N., Ren, J., Peters, T.M.: Rapid registration of multimodal images using a reduced number of voxels procedures. In: SPIE Medical Imaging, vol. 6141, p. 34756 (2006)
6. Ma, Y.L., Penney, G.P., Rinaldi, C.A., Cooklin, M., Razavi, R., Rhode, K.S.: Echocardiography to magnetic resonance image registration for use in image-guided cardiac catheterization procedures. Phys. Med. Biol. **54**, 5039–5055 (2009)
7. Savi, A., Gilardi, M.C., Rizzo, G., Pepi, M., Landoni, C., Rossetti, C., Lucignani, G., Bartorelli, A., Fazio, F.: Spatial registration of echocardiographic and positron emission tomographic heart studies. Eur. J. Nucl. Med. **22**(3), 243–247 (1995)
8. Sinha, S., Sinha, U., Czernin, J., Porenta, G., Schelbert, H.: Noninvasive assessment of myocardial perfusion and metabolism: feasibility of registering gated MR and PET images. AJR Am. J. Roentgenol. **164**(2), 301–307 (1995)
9. Zhuang, X.: Challenges and methodologies of fully automatic whole heart segmentation: a review. J. Healthc. Eng. **3**, 371–407 (2013)
10. Spreeuwers, L., Bangma, S., Meerwaldt, R., Vonken, E., Breeuwer, M.: Detection of trabeculae and papillary muscles in cardiac MR images. Comput. Cardiol., 415–418 (2005)
11. Gao, M., Chen, C., Zhang, S., Qian, Z., Metaxas, D., Axel, L.: Segmenting the papillary muscles and the trabeculae from high resolution cardiac CT through restoration of topological handles. In: Gee, J.C., Joshi, S., Pohl, K.M., Wells, W.M., Zöllei, L. (eds.) IPMI 2013. LNCS, vol. 7917, pp. 184–195. Springer, Heidelberg (2013)
12. Zuluaga, M.A., Cardoso, M.J., Modat, M., Ourselin, S.: Multi-atlas propagation whole heart segmentation from MRI and CTA using a local normalised correlation coefficient criterion. In: Ourselin, S., Rueckert, D., Smith, N. (eds.) FIMH 2013. LNCS, vol. 7945, pp. 174–181. Springer, Heidelberg (2013)
13. Uribe, S., Tangchaoren, T., Parish, V., Wolf, I., Razavi, R., Greil, G., Schaeffter, T.: Volumetric cardiac quantification by using 3D dual-phase whole-heart MR imaging1. Radiology **248**, 606–614 (2008)
14. Yushkevich, P.A., Piven, J., Cody Hazlett, H., Gimpel Smith, R., Ho, S., Gee, J.C., Gerig, G.: User-guided 3D active contour segmentation of anatomical structures: significantly improved efficiency and reliability. Neuroimage **31**(3), 1116–1128 (2006)
15. Petitjean, C., Zuluaga, M.A., Bai, W., Dacher, J.N., Grosgeorge, D., Caudron, J., Ruan, S., Ayed, I.B., Cardoso, M.J., Chen, H.C., Jimenez-Carretero, D., Ledesma-Carbayo, M.J., Davatzikos, C., Doshi, J., Erus, G., Maier, O.M., Nambakhsh, C.M., Ou, Y., Ourselin, S., Peng, C.W., Peters, N.S., Peters, T.M., Rajchl, M., Rueckert, D., Santos, A., Shi, W., Wang, C.W., Wang, H., Yuan, J.: Right ventricle segmentation from cardiac MRI: a collation study. Med. Image Anal. **19**(1), 187–202 (2015)

16. Tobón-Gómez, C., Geers, A., Peters, J., Weese, J., Pinto, K., Karim, R., Ammar, M., Daoudi, A., Margeta, J., Sandoval, Z., Stender, B., Zheng, Y., Zuluaga, M.A., Betancur, J., Ayache, N., Chikh, M.A., Dillenseger, J.L., Mahmoudi, S., Kelm, B.M., Ourselin, S., Schlaefer, A., Schaeffter, T., Razavi, R., Rhode, K.: Benchmark for algorithms segmenting the left atrium from 3D CT and MRI datasets. IEEE Trans. Med. Imaging **34** (2015)

17. Cardoso, M., Leung, K., Modat, M., Keihaninejad, S., Cash, D., Barnes, J., Fox, N., Ourselin, S.: STEPS: similarity and truth estimation for propagated segmentations and its application to hippocampal segmentation and brain parcelation. Med. Image Anal. **17**(6), 671–684 (2013)

Electrophysiology Model for a Human Heart with Ischemic Scar and Realistic Purkinje Network

Toni Lassila[1]($\boxtimes$), Matthias Lange[1], Antonio R. Porras Perez[2], Karim Lekadir[2], Xènia Albà[2], Gemma Piella[2], and Alejandro F. Frangi[1]

[1] Department of Electronic and Electrical Engineering,
Centre for Computational Imaging and Simulation Technologies
in Biomedicine (CISTIB), The University of Sheffield, Sheffield, UK
`t.lassila@sheffield.ac.uk`
[2] Department of Information and Communications Technologies,
Centre for Computational Imaging and Simulation Technologies
in Biomedicine (CISTIB), Universitat Pompeu Fabra, Barcelona, Spain

Abstract. The role of Purkinje fibres in the onset of arrhythmias is controversial and computer simulations may shed light on possible arrhythmic mechanisms involving the Purkinje fibres. However, few computational modelling studies currently include a detailed Purkinje network as part of the model. We present a coupled Purkinje-myocardium electrophysiology model that includes an explicit model for the ischemic scar plus a detailed Purkinje network, and compare simulated activation times to those obtained by electro-anatomical mapping in vivo during sinus rhythm pacing. The results illustrate the importance of using sufficiently dense Purkinje networks in patient-specific studies to capture correctly the myocardial early activation that may be influenced by surviving Purkinje fibres in the infarct region.

1 Introduction

Personalised computational electrophysiology (EP) models are increasingly improving in the level of anatomical and physiological detail, and their personalisation, so as to hold the promise of enabling personalised planning of ablation targets in terminating ventricular tachycardias (VT). There is some evidence that certain type of arrhythmias may be triggered by ectopic beats originating from Purkinje fibre automaticity during acute myocardial infarction [2]. Until recently, however, most EP simulations have neglected the effect of the Purkinje network (PN) or used very coarse networks. Thus the first step towards more complete modelling of ventricular tachycardia (VT) is to develop realistic models of coupled myocardium-Purkinje whole-heart models, and to validate them against physiological measurements of activation patterns.

We present a computational pipeline for human EP modelling with: (i) a PN model based on a rule-based algorithm for generating the network and a set of

© Springer International Publishing Switzerland 2016
O. Camara et al. (Eds.): STACOM 2015, LNCS 9534, pp. 90–97, 2016.
DOI: 10.1007/978-3-319-28712-6_10

cable equations on line segments coupled together by the gap junction resistance model [16]; (ii) a myocardium model based on the monodomain approximation and the left ventricular (LV) action potential (AP) model of Bueno-Orovio et al. [3]; and (iii) electrical remodelling in the scar/borderzone by fitting the model of Bueno-Orovio et al. to a modified ten Tusscher-Panfilov 2006 - model [14].

We then compare the model predictions against electro-anatomical mapping (EAM) data consisting of endocardial activation times in a patient with extensive myocardial scarring. The EAM data is projected onto the simulated LV geometry to compare the local activation times (LAT). Results are given for varying levels of Purkinje-muscle junction (PMJ) density.

2   Models for Cardiac Electrophysiology

A standard monodomain approximation for myocardial tissue is used:

$$\chi \left[c_m \frac{\partial u}{\partial t} + i_{ion}, (u, v, r, s) - i_{app}(t) \right] = \nabla \cdot (\sigma \nabla u), \qquad (1)$$

where the ionic current, $i_{ion} = i_{fi} + i_{si} + i_{so}$, consists of the fast/slow inward, and slow outward currents respectively, which are gated by the internal membrane variables v, r, s as in Bueno-Orovio et al. 2008 [3]. The conductivity tensor in (1) depends on a spatially varying parameter γ s.t. $\sigma = (1 - \gamma_i) [\sigma_t I + (\sigma_l - \sigma_t) f_0 \otimes f_0]$. To account for structural remodelling under chronic myocardial infarction, the conduction velocity (CV) in the deep scar and its surrounding border zone are typically modified. As first approximation the membrane model is turned off and the CV is set to zero throughout the deep scar region. However, experimental evidence on rabbits [17] indicates greatly reduced conductivity (10 % of normal CV) in the borderzone surrounding the scar, but close to normal conductivity in the infarcted region (50 % of normal CV), and in some cases even the possibility to stimulate the infarcted region. Accordingly, we used $\gamma_{healthy} = 0$, $\gamma_{border} = 0.97$, and $\gamma_{scar} = 0.75$, and the longitudinal and transversal conductivities are $\sigma_l = 1.5 \, kOhm^{-1}cm^{-1}$, $\sigma_t = 0.6 \, kOhm^{-1}cm^{-1}$. This corresponds to reducing the conduction velocity to 8 % in the borderzone and 44 % in the scar region. Fibre dispersion is not considered.

The effects of ischemia include hyperkalemia, changes in the fast Na^+ and L-type Ca^{2+} channels, hypoxia, and acidosis. These effects can be modelled in the ten Tusscher-Panfilov 2006 -model by adding an extra ATP-sensitive K^+ current, as was done in [6]. The extracellular potassium concentrations are kept at their normal levels to avoid elevated resting potentials. The modified parameters describing mild and severe ischemia are taken from [8].

Once the ten Tusscher-Panfilov 2006 -model has been extended, APs from rest are extracted. A subset of 7 parameters in the Bueno-Orovio et al. -model is selected for optimisation. A curve-fitting problem for the AP is solved and parameters that do not change from their reference values are replaced by educated choice. The process is repeated until an accurate replication of the AP shape is obtained. The final values of the modified parameters are (borderzone/scar): k_w = 65.0356/65.0356, τ_{o1} = 6.3196/5.3307, τ_{so1} = 56.6591/56.1802, τ_{so2} = 1.0809/1.5291, k_{so} = 2.2695/2.4552, τ_{s2} = 7.3099/7.6184, k_s = 5.6456/5.7472.

The PN is modelled as a network of line segments (with loops) with the model of Vigmond et al. [16]. We use the Di Francesco-Noble [4] membrane model with standard parameters for the PN. The conductivity and membrane model of the PN remains unchanged in the borderzone and scar regions. The numerical algorithm used for the PN is described in more detail in [7]. The connection between the PN and the myocardium is modelled using a coupled resistor and distributed current source -model that captures the 3–5 ms delay in orthodromic propagation. We do not consider the antidromic conduction back into the PN in this work.

3   Computational Electrophysiology Model Generation

LV segmentation is performed from cardiac MRI with delayed enhancement (DE-MRI) as described in [12]. The segmentation thresholds have been previously optimized using EAM data in [1,5]. These thresholds have been used to successfully identify borderzone conducting channels during catheter ablation. After projecting the intensity values to a surface mesh segmentation of the LV, 4,000 radial basis function interpolation sites are randomly seeded on the endo- and epicardial surfaces respectively. The intensity values are interpolated using inverse multi-quadric shape functions and used to choose the appropriate membrane model parameters using the same criterion as in [5] that intensity above >60 % of maximum is considered scar, while <40 % of the maximum is considered healthy tissue – everything in between is considered borderzone.

Rule-based Poisson interpolation is applied to obtain fibre orientations. The LV centreline is identified automatically and a linearly graded fibre orientation from −41° on the endocardium to +60° on the epicardium is obtained. Three levels of PNs of increasing density (166 PMJs in the low-density case, 756 PMJs in the mid-density case, and 1,296 PMJs in the high-density case) are generated to test the impact of PMJ density on the activation pattern. A 2 cm area below the basal cut-plane contains no PMJs as reported in literature. The resulting PN is fitted to the endocardium, but is not modified according to the LAT observed in the EAM. While methods exist [10,11,15] to fit the PMJ distribution to patient-specific observations of endocardial LAT, the danger of over- fitting the model to available data exists. Increasing the number of PMJs allows fitting of the LAT with arbitrary accuracy at least in the regions where the PN is present, but without necessarily providing meaningful information about the actual morphology of the PN. A crude fitting algorithm may, for example, prefer to eliminate the PN completely from the infarct scar region in order to match the LAT, which is not supported by the evidence of the PN surviving in the infarct core with prolonged action-potential duration and enhanced automaticity [9]. We therefore rely on the observations of [15] that even without personalising the PMJ locations, sufficiently dense tentative PNs can predict LAT with reasonable accuracy.

4   Results

The EAM dataset was obtained with the CARTO system (Biosense Webster, Haifa, Israel) and consisted of bipolar/unipolar voltages, LAT, and position of each catheter point on or near the endocardium. Measurements were made with a tetrapolar diagnostic catheter (Thermocool, Navistar, Biosense Webster) in a total of 671 locations on the LV endocardium and around the mitral annulus. After having the segmentation from DE-MR, this was imported into CARTO and registration was done manually using the CARTO software during the intervention. The experimental methodology is described in more detail in [12]. The LV had considerable post-infarction myocardial scarring several days after the initial infarct (see Fig. 1). Previous studies [5,13] have shown a moderate correlation between the scar regions obtained from EAM by bipolar voltage thresholds (<0.5 mV for the scar and 0.5–1.5 mV for the borderzone) and the DE-MRI-derived endocardial scar regions, so that we treated the DE-MRI-derived scar regions as having been previously validated. Simulations were run for both the cases where the scar region was assumed to be nonexcitable tissue (not shown) and excitable tissue with the parameters identified by the nonlinear fitting procedure. While the subject's LV was heavily scarred both transmurally and apex-to-base on the lateral side, the EAM did confirm slow CV but not propagation failure in the scar regions. Thus the case of nonexcitable scar tissue was rejected due to insufficient activation of the LV scar region compared to the EAM results.

Figure 2 shows the LAT measured from EAM and interpolated onto the lateral endocardium (left) compared with the simulated LAT (right). Despite no personalisation being performed on the myofibre orientation nor on the PN, correspondence is good at the apex and mid-wall. The largest difference in LAT

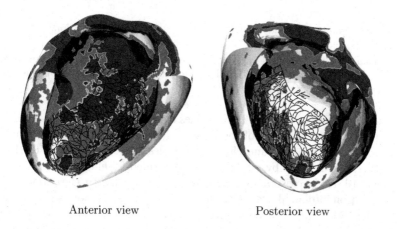

| Anterior view | Posterior view |

Fig. 1. Scar and its borderzone identified from DE-MRI according to the criteria in [5]. Color scheme indicates red for deep scar, blue for borderzone, and white for healthy myocardium. Tentative PN superimposed for reference. Large percentage of PMJs in the posterolateral free-wall lie in the deep scar region (Color figure online).

takes place near the basal regions. Figure 3 shows the bullseye plot of mean LAT on each of the 17 AHA segments for the three different densities of PNs. As coverage improves, the LAT more closely corresponds to timings measured by EAM. The largest differences can again be observed at the basal area, which we explain as follows. In the EAM data there are some catheter locations that are clustered near the aortic valve and the mitral annulus. Projecting the data from these points onto the truncated LV surface may produce spurious data that make the recorded basal LAT unreliable. We do not consider this a serious problem, as the basolateral region is known to activate last and therefore plays a lesser role in the induction of VT.

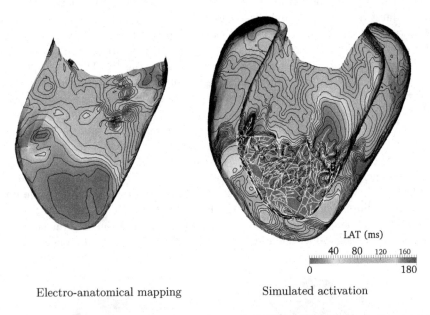

LAT (ms)

40   80   120   160

0   180

Electro-anatomical mapping   Simulated activation

Fig. 2. The LAT on the septal endocardium for EAM (left) and simulation (right). Isochrones of LAT present every 10 ms. High-density PN superimposed on the right.

To analyse more closely the discrepancies observed in certain AHA segments, we present in Fig. 4 a box plot of the LAT in the EAM (top) and the simulation (bottom). Segment medians and 25–75 percentiles are represented by the boxes, while outliers are denoted by red crosses (jitter added for enhanced readability). In segments 10–17 the existence of endocardial scarring divides the surface points in the simulation into an almost bimodal distribution – some points get activated early by the PMJs (denoted by points falling around the median) while others get activated late due to slow propagation in the deep scar region (the outliers). Comparing against the EAM we find that the median LAT in the EAM measurements is closer to the LAT of the simulation outliers, which may be either because the catheter measurements were not able to measure the PMJ-induced activation, or because the PMJs in the scar region were not activated. A similar

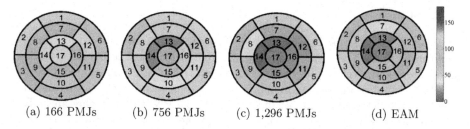

(a) 166 PMJs   (b) 756 PMJs   (c) 1,296 PMJs   (d) EAM

Fig. 3. Mean endocardial LAT [ms] in the 17 AHA segments for the simulation using low, mid or high-density PN (from left to right), compared to the EAM (far right).

situation exists in segments 3–5. Interestingly, in this case also the EAM measurements possess outliers but in the early activation region, which appears to indicate that at least some of the PMJ-induced activation was picked up by the catheter measurements. In the mid anterior segments without any scarring (7–9) the confidence intervals are roughly overlapping.

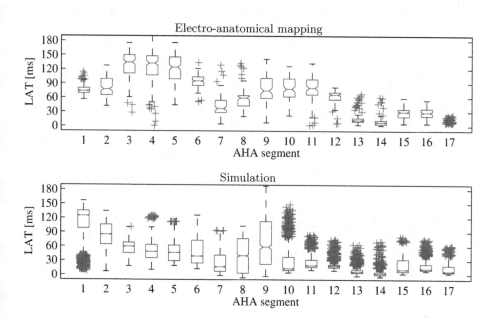

Fig. 4. Box plots of LAT for EAM (top) and simulation (bottom) grouped by AHA segment. Red crosses denote outliers that do not fall within the confidence intervals. The simulated LAT exhibits a strongly bimodal distribution in segments with scarring (Color figure online).

5   Discussion

The importance of the Purkinje fibre network in the genesis of ventricular arrhythmias and VT is still a subject of debate in the clinical community. Consequently, few computer studies have focused on its effect or even included it in the models. Computational VT inducibility studies tend to mimic the experimental protocols, i.e. external pacing scenarios, where the PN does not play an active role. We propose that better understanding of the role and function of the PN in arrhythmias is important also in the sinus rhythm case, and to this end the first step is to construct robust and validated models of pathological ventricular activation including the effects of the PN.

We presented a pipeline for EP simulations on a patient-specific LV geometry with ischemic myocardial scarring and a detailed Purkinje network for initial activation under sinus rhythm. Even without personalising the PN or myofibre directions, reasonably good agreement between simulated and experimental LAT was obtained, provided that the PMJ coverage was dense enough. Excitable myocytes had to be modelled in the myocardial scar to obtain correspondence between EAM and simulation. There may exist a viable sub-endocardial layer 3–5 cells deep (due to oxygen diffusion from the blood pool) that allows conduction to take place in the scar, explaining the survival of the Purkinje fibres.

Our model has certain limitations. It does not account for transmural variations in the myocardial cells nor variations in the AP of the PN in ischemia; hence the validation centred mainly on the endocardial LAT. To study the transmural propagation, either an EAM study with epicardial LAT needs to be performed, or an extension to the bidomain model should be made, in order to validate against the ECG. In order to model left bundle branch block (a typical comorbidity in the myocardial infarction cases we observed), the model should also be extended to include the right ventricle with corresponding validation by EAM. Further validation on multiple patient-specific instances is also needed.

Acknowledgement. This research has been partially funded by the Industrial and Technological Development Center (CDTI) under the CENIT-cvREMOD program. The work of A.R. Porras and X. Albà was supported by the Spanish Government under FPU grant. A.F. Frangi was partially funded by the ICREA-Academia program. Clinical data used in this study was provided by A. Berruezo, D. Andreu, J. Fernández-Armenta, and M. Sitges from the Hospital Clinic of Barcelona.

References

1. Andreu, D., Berruezo, A., Ortiz-Pérez, J., Silva, E., Mont, L., Borràs, R., de Caralt, T., Perea, R., Fernández-Armenta, J., Zeljko, H., et al.: Integration of 3D electroanatomic maps and magnetic resonance scar characterization into the navigation system to guide ventricular tachycardia ablation. Circ. Arrhythm. Electrophysiol. **4**(5), 674–683 (2011)
2. Bogun, F., Good, E., Reich, S., Elmouchi, D., Igic, P., Tschopp, D., Dey, S., Wimmer, A., Jongnarangsin, K., Oral, H., et al.: Role of Purkinje fibers in post-infarction ventricular tachycardia. J. Am. Coll. Cardiol. **48**(12), 2500–2507 (2006)

3. Bueno-Orovio, A., Cherry, E.M., Fenton, F.H.: Minimal model for human ventricular action potentials in tissue. J. Theor. Biol. **253**(3), 544–560 (2008)
4. DiFrancesco, D., Noble, D.: A model of cardiac electrical activity incorporating ionic pumps and concentration changes. Phil. Trans. R. Soc. B **307**(1133), 353–398 (1985)
5. Fernández-Armenta, J., Berruezo, A., Andreu, D., Camara, O., Silva, E., Serra, L., Barbarito, V., et al.: Three-dimensional architecture of scar and conducting channels based on high resolution CE-CMR insights for ventricular tachycardia ablation. Circ. Arrhythm. Electrophysiol. **6**(3), 528–537 (2013)
6. Heidenreich, E., Rodríguez, J., Doblaré, M., Trénor, B., Ferrero, J.: Electrical propagation patterns in a 3D regionally ischemic human heart: a simulation study. IEEE Comput. Cardiol., 665–668 (2009)
7. Lange, M., Palamara, S., Lassila, T., Vergara, C., Quarteroni, A., Frangi, A.F.: Efficient numerical schemes for computing cardiac electrical activation over realistic Purkinje networks: method and verification. In: van Assen, H., Bovendeerd, P., Delhaas, T. (eds.) FIMH 2015. LNCS, vol. 9126, pp. 430–438. Springer, Heidelberg (2015)
8. Lu, W., Wang, K., Zhang, H., Zuo, W.: Simulation of ECG under ischemic condition in human ventricular tissue. IEEE Comput. Cardiol. **37**, 185–188 (2010)
9. Nattel, S., Maguy, A., Le Bouter, S., Yeh, Y.H.: Arrhythmogenic ion-channel remodeling in the heart: heart failure, myocardial infarction, and atrial fibrillation. Physiol. Rev. **87**(2), 425–456 (2007)
10. Palamara, S., Vergara, C., Catanzariti, D., Faggiano, E., Pangrazzi, C., Centonze, M., Nobile, F., Maines, M., Quarteroni, A.: Computational generation of the Purkinje network driven by clinical measurements: the case of pathological propagations. Int. J. Numer. Methods Biomed. Engr. **30**(12), 1558–1577 (2014)
11. Palamara, S., Vergara, C., Faggiano, E., Nobile, F.: An effective algorithm for the generation of patient-specific Purkinje networks in computational electrocardiology. J. Comp. Phys. **283**, 495–517 (2015)
12. Porras, A., Piella, G., Berruezo, A., Fernández-Armenta, J., Frangi, A.: Pre-to intra-operative data fusion framework for multimodal characterization of myocardial scar tissue. IEEE J. Transl. Eng. Health Med. 2 (2015)
13. Porras, A., Piella, G., Berruezo, A., Hoogendoorn, C., Andreu, D., Fernandez-Armenta, J., Sitges, M., Frangi, A.: Interventional endocardial motion estimation from electroanatomical mapping data: application to scar characterization. IEEE Trans. Biomed. Eng. **60**(5), 1217–1224 (2013)
14. ten Tusscher, K.H., Panfilov, A.V.: Alternans and spiral breakup in a human ventricular tissue model. Am. J. Physiol. Heart C. **291**(3), H1088–H1100 (2006)
15. Vergara, C., Palamara, S., Catanzariti, D., Nobile, F., Faggiano, E., Pangrazzi, C., Centonze, M., Maines, M., Quarteroni, A., Vergara, G.: Patient-specific generation of the Purkinje network driven by clinical measurements of a normal propagation. Med. Bio. Eng. Comput. **52**(10), 813–826 (2014)
16. Vigmond, E., Clements, C.: Construction of a computer model to investigate sawtooth effects in the Purkinje system. IEEE Trans. Biomed. Eng. **54**(3), 389–399 (2007)
17. Walker, N., Burton, F., Kettlewell, S., Smith, G., Cobbe, S.: Mapping of epicardial activation in a rabbit model of chronic myocardial infarction. J. Cardiovasc. Electrophysiol. **18**(8), 862–868 (2007)

Patient Metadata-Constrained Shape Models for Cardiac Image Segmentation

Marco Pereañez[1](✉), Karim Lekadir[1], Xenia Albà[1], Pau Medrano-Gracia[2], Alistair A. Young[2], and Alejandro Frangi[3]

[1] Center for Computational Imaging and Simulation Technologies
in Biomedicine (CISTIB), Universitat Pompeu Fabra, Barcelona, Spain
marco.pereanez@upf.edu
[2] Department of Anatomy with Radiology, University of Auckland,
Auckland, New Zealand
[3] Center for Computational Imaging and Simulation Technologies
in Biomedicine (CISTIB), University of Sheffield, Sheffield, UK

Abstract. Patient metadata such as demographic information and cardio vascular disease (CVD) indicators are valuable data readily available in clinical practice. This information can be used to inform the construction of customized statistical shape models fitting the patient's unique characteristics. However, to the best of our knowledge, no studies have reported using these types of metadata in the construction of shape models for image segmentation. In this paper, we propose the use of a conditional model framework to include these patient metadata in the construction of a personalized shape model and evaluate its effect on image segmentation. Our validation on a dataset of 250 asymptomatic cardiac MR images shows an average segmentation improvement of 7 % and in some cases up to 30 % over a conventional PCA-based framework. These results show the potential of our technique for improved shape analysis.

1 Introduction

Cardiac segmentation is a prerequisite for a number of important clinical applications ranging from the relatively simple computation of ejection fraction (EF), to understanding disease progression through shape analysis in longitudinal studies, to more complex tasks, such as, simulating cardio-vascular function and electrophysiology for treatment planning and intervention. All of these tasks require accurate segmentation of the cardiac structure in order to obtain reliable and meaningful outputs.

Segmentation of cardiac structures, however, remains a challenging task due to the high geometric complexity of the organ, as well as image inhomogeneities. To overcome these problems, statistical shape model-based methods have been widely adopted due to their ability to simplify shape complexity and overcome noisy image information through the model fitting process. Nevertheless, these

© Springer International Publishing Switzerland 2016
O. Camara et al. (Eds.): STACOM 2015, LNCS 9534, pp. 98–107, 2016.
DOI: 10.1007/978-3-319-28712-6_11

model-based techniques have traditionally only focused on the use of shape information for the construction of models and do not include other potentially useful non-image derived information typically found on a patient's clinical chart.

In our review of the literature we found a study by Wolz et al. [10] that reports using both patient and image metadata to enhance their manifold learning technique for the purpose of brain image classification. In another study, Blanc et al. [2] use what they refer to as surrogate variables of the femur bone i.e., different anatomical lengths and angles within the bone and patient information, to further constrain the shape space of a PCA derived model and study their influence. Grbić et al. [6] use landmark derived features to build a patient specific model with a reduced set of shapes for image segmentation. Finally, Medrano-Gracia et al. [7] quantify and show significant morphological differences in asymptomatic cardiac shape between different demographic and risk factor sub-groups. They do this by performing PCA on the sub-groups, and evaluating the statistical significance of differences between their principal modes of variation. Although all of these works address the issue of including other non-image data in the analysis of shape, none of them use patient-metadata for cardiac segmentation, which is the focus of this paper.

In this paper, we propose the use of a conditional shape model framework [8] for the definition of a shape distribution constrained by demographic data and CVD indicators and apply it to cardiac image segmentation. We validate our framework by comparing the segmentation accuracy of our method with that of a standard PCA-based model.

The remainder of this paper is organized as follows: In Sect. 2, we describe the details regarding model construction and segmentation. In Sect. 3, we present the obtained segmentation results and comparison to the standard PCA-based model. Finally, conclusions are drawn in Sect. 4.

2   Method

This section describes the statistical modeling of the probability distribution of shape conditioned on metadata, i.e. $P(\mathbf{x}|\mathbf{m}_j)$. More specifically, we would like to compute a Point Distribution Model (PDM) for shapes $\mathbf{x}_i$ based on their conditional relationship with each metadata field $\mathbf{m}_j$, that is, a mean $\bar{\mathbf{x}}_{\mathbf{m}_j}$, and covariance matrix $\boldsymbol{\Sigma}_{\mathbf{x}|\mathbf{m}_j}$. Subsequently, we combine these conditional PDMs into one unified PDM that accounts for all shape-metadata relationships. Lastly, we describe the image feature search and model fitting process.

Our method consists of four main steps:

1. **Metadata-Constrained Allowable Domain:** Given a dataset of shape vectors $\mathbf{x}_i$, $i = 1, ..., N$ obtained from previously segmented images, and their corresponding metadata fields $\mathbf{m}_{i,j}$, $j = 1, ..., M$, we compute a set of eigenspaces $E_j = \{\boldsymbol{\Phi}, \boldsymbol{\Lambda}_j\}$ that describe the allowable shape space for shapes $\mathbf{x}_i$ conditioned on metadata $\mathbf{m}_{i,j}$. To train these models, we use the definitions of multivariate conditional distributions described in Sect. 2.1.

2. **Metadata-Constrained Mean Shape:** Based on a new patient's metadata $\mathbf{m}_j^{new}$, we compute M new mean shape estimates $\bar{\mathbf{x}}_{\mathbf{m}_j}$, and combine them to obtain the final model estimate $\bar{\mathbf{x}}_c$ (see Sect. 2.2).
3. **Metadata Constraints Combination:** The final allowable domain $\boldsymbol{\Lambda}_c$ is computed as the intersecting space from the different metadata-constrained variances as estimated in step 1, centered on their corresponding mean estimates $\bar{\mathbf{x}}_{\mathbf{m}_j}$ computed on step 2 (see Sect. 2.3).
4. **Application to Image Search:** We use the obtained metadata constrained PDM to guide the image segmentation of a new patient's image volume. We use the Sparse Active Shape Models (SPASM) framework [9] to perform the cardiac image segmentation in this paper (see Sect. 2.4).

2.1 Metadata-Constrained Allowable Domain

Let us define an augmented shape data matrix $\mathbf{D}$ by appending metadata values $\mathbf{m}_{i,j}$ to the last index of shape vectors $\mathbf{x}_i$ (Eq. 1).

$$\mathbf{D} = \left[\left\{ \begin{matrix} \mathbf{x}_1 \\ \mathbf{m}_{1,j} \end{matrix} \right\}, \ldots, \left\{ \begin{matrix} \mathbf{x}_N \\ \mathbf{m}_{N,j} \end{matrix} \right\} \right] \tag{1}$$

Using $\mathbf{D}$ we compute the block covariance matrix $\boldsymbol{\Sigma}_{\mathbf{DD}}$ as shown on Eq. 2.

$$\boldsymbol{\Sigma}_{\mathbf{DD}} = \begin{bmatrix} \boldsymbol{\Sigma}_{\mathbf{xx}} & \boldsymbol{\Sigma}_{\mathbf{xm}_j} \\ \boldsymbol{\Sigma}_{\mathbf{xm}_j}^T & \boldsymbol{\Sigma}_{\mathbf{m}_j\mathbf{m}_j} \end{bmatrix}. \tag{2}$$

The conditional covariance estimates that relate shape in $\mathbf{x}_i$, and metadata $\mathbf{m}_j$ are calculated using Eq. 3.

$$\boldsymbol{\Sigma}_{\mathbf{x}|\mathbf{m}_j} = \boldsymbol{\Sigma}_{\mathbf{xx}} - \boldsymbol{\Sigma}_{\mathbf{xm}_j} \boldsymbol{\Sigma}_{\mathbf{m}_j\mathbf{m}_j}^{-1} \boldsymbol{\Sigma}_{\mathbf{xm}_j}^T. \tag{3}$$

The covariance matrices in Eq. 3 are obtained from the block covariance matrix in Eq. 2. $\boldsymbol{\Sigma}_{\mathbf{xm}_j} \boldsymbol{\Sigma}_{\mathbf{m}_j\mathbf{m}_j}^{-1}$ are the regression coefficients that model the relationship between shape and the metadata fields. These coefficients are stored and used to compute the final mean shape estimate of the model in the next section.

Since for N models we have to perform N eigendecompositions on relatively large covariance matrices $\boldsymbol{\Sigma}_{\mathbf{x}|\mathbf{m}_j}$, we choose to reduce the dimensionality of the problem by working with parametric shape vectors $\mathbf{b}_i = \boldsymbol{\Phi}^T(\mathbf{x}_i - \bar{\mathbf{x}})$ through eigendecomposition of $\boldsymbol{\Sigma}_{\mathbf{xx}}$, rather than 3D shape vectors $\mathbf{x}_i$. We retained 98% of variance after eigendecomposition, which, depending on the size of the training set is accounted for by 20 to 30 modes of variation. With this new representation, Eq. 2 is replaced by Eq. 4,

$$\boldsymbol{\Sigma}_{\mathbf{DD}}^{(b)} = \begin{bmatrix} \boldsymbol{\Lambda}_{\mathbf{bb}} & \boldsymbol{\Sigma}_{\mathbf{bm}_j} \\ \boldsymbol{\Sigma}_{\mathbf{bm}_j}^T & \boldsymbol{\Sigma}_{\mathbf{m}_j\mathbf{m}_j} \end{bmatrix} \tag{4}$$

where $\boldsymbol{\Lambda}_{\mathbf{bb}}$ are the eigenvalues of $\boldsymbol{\Sigma}_{\mathbf{xx}}$, and subindex $\mathbf{b}$ indicates parametric shape.

Similarly, Eq. 3 is replaced by Eq. 5,

$$\mathbf{\Lambda}_{\mathbf{m}_j} = \mathbf{\Lambda}_{\mathbf{bb}} - \mathbf{\Sigma}_{\mathbf{bm}_j} \mathbf{\Sigma}^{-1}_{\mathbf{m}_j \mathbf{m}_j} \mathbf{\Sigma}^T_{\mathbf{bm}_j}, \tag{5}$$

where $\mathbf{\Lambda}_{\mathbf{m}_j}$ is a subset of the variance in $\mathbf{\Lambda}_{\mathbf{bb}}$, and has the same coordinate system $\mathbf{\Phi}$ that represents parametric shapes $\mathbf{b}_i$.

Using Eqs. 4 and 5 we obtain M eigenvalue matrices $\mathbf{\Lambda}_{\mathbf{m}_j}$ that represent the conditional shape variability of $\mathbf{x}_i$ with respect to each metadata field $\mathbf{m}_j$.

Thus far, we have a coordinate system $\mathbf{\Phi}$ and M conditional variance matrices $\mathbf{\Lambda}_{\mathbf{b}|\mathbf{m}_j}$. However, we still need to compute M corresponding conditional mean vectors $\bar{\mathbf{b}}_{\mathbf{m}_j}$, to which $\mathbf{\Lambda}_{\mathbf{b}|\mathbf{m}_j}$ are centered, and combine these models into a unique PDM that encodes all conditional relationships between shape and metadata.

2.2 Metadata-Constrained Mean Shape

In order to compute the final model's mean shape, we first need to compute M mean estimates $\bar{\mathbf{b}}_{\mathbf{m}_j}$ using the regression coefficients $\mathbf{\Sigma}_{\mathbf{bm}_j} \mathbf{\Sigma}^{-1}_{\mathbf{m}_j \mathbf{m}_j}$ obtained in Sect. 2.1. Using these coefficients, and the definitions of multivariate conditional normal distributions, we obtain M conditional mean estimates based on each metadata field (Eq. 6).

$$\bar{\mathbf{b}}_{\mathbf{m}_j} = \mathbf{\Sigma}_{\mathbf{bm}j} \mathbf{\Sigma}^{-1}_{\mathbf{m}_j \mathbf{m}_j} (\mathbf{m}^{new}_j - \bar{\mathbf{m}}_j) \tag{6}$$

Notice that in Eq. 6, $\mathbf{m}^{new}_j$ is the jth metadata field of a new subject for whom shape is unknown.

The question then becomes how to combine these mean shape estimates into the final mean. Given that not all metadata are good predictors of shape, we weigh each mean estimate proportionally to the degree of correlation between shape and the different metadata fields (Eq. 7),

$$w_j = \frac{\rho_{\mathbf{b}_i \mathbf{m}_j}}{\sum \rho_{\mathbf{b}_i \mathbf{m}_j}} \tag{7}$$

where $\rho_{\mathbf{x}_i \mathbf{m}_j}$ is the correlation coefficient between shape and each metadata field.

The final parametric mean estimate $\bar{\mathbf{b}}$ is a weighted average of the previously obtained mean estimates $\bar{\mathbf{b}}_{\mathbf{m}_j}$ (Eq. 8). The final mean shape in 3D space is recovered using Eq. 9. We denote the final conditional model parameters with subindex c.

$$\bar{\mathbf{b}} = \sum_{j=1}^{M} \bar{\mathbf{b}}_{\mathbf{m}_j} w_j \tag{8}$$

$$\bar{\mathbf{x}}_c = \bar{\mathbf{x}} + \mathbf{\Phi}\bar{\mathbf{b}} \tag{9}$$

2.3   Metadata Constraints Combination

The variance associated to the final mean, $\bar{\mathbf{x}}_c$, is computed by centering the previously obtained eigenvalue matrices $\mathbf{\Lambda}_{\mathbf{m}_j}$ at their corresponding mean estimates $\bar{\mathbf{b}}_{\mathbf{m}_j}$, and calculating the overlapping space between all eigenspaces $E_j = \{\mathbf{\Phi}, \mathbf{\Lambda}_{\mathbf{m}_j}\}$. Equation 10 describes the intersecting space, where $\lambda_{\mathbf{m}_j}$ are the diagonal entries of eigenvalue matices $\mathbf{\Lambda}_{\mathbf{m}_j}$.

$$\lambda_c = \frac{1}{2}\left\{\min_j(\bar{\mathbf{b}}_{\mathbf{m}_j} + \lambda_{\mathbf{m}_j}) + |\max_j(\bar{\mathbf{b}}_{\mathbf{m}_j} - \lambda_{\mathbf{m}_j})|\right\} \tag{10}$$

By assembling a diagonal matrix with the entries of λ_c, we obtain the final eigenvalue matrix $\mathbf{\Lambda}_c$ describing the conditional variability of shapes $\mathbf{x}_i$ given metadata $\mathbf{m}_j$. The final PDM described in Eq. 11 will be used to constrain image segmentation in the next section.

$$\Omega_{\mathbf{x}|\mathbf{m}} = (\bar{\mathbf{x}}_c, \mathbf{\Phi}, \mathbf{\Lambda}_c) \tag{11}$$

2.4   Application to Image Search

Boundary Detection. Image boundaries were detected by minimizing the Mahalanobis distance between a profile of grey levels $\mathbf{g}$ sampled from each landmark of the current shape estimate, and the mean profile from the training set $\bar{\mathbf{g}}$. The appearance model for each landmark is trained by computing the mean $\bar{\mathbf{g}}$, and covariance matrix $\mathbf{\Sigma}_{\mathbf{gg}}$, for the profiles of corresponding landmarks across the training set. Landmark profiles $\mathbf{g}$ are sampled by projecting a normal vector to the shape's surface onto the image slice closest to that landmark. Subsequently, the Mahalanobis distance between every point in the model and the profile is computed. Finally, the landmark is displaced to the location that minimizes the distance on Eq. 12.

$$D(\mathbf{g}) = \sqrt{(\mathbf{g} - \bar{\mathbf{g}})^T \mathbf{\Sigma}_{\mathbf{gg}}^{-1}(\mathbf{g} - \bar{\mathbf{g}})} \tag{12}$$

Shape Model Fitting. After the landmark displacement procedure described in the previous section, the new feature points need to be constrained to ensure they constitute a valid shape (described by our PDM). We do this following a standard procedure [3] to find the pose and shape parameters that best fit the new feature points. Let us assume we wish to fit a new model instance $\tilde{\mathbf{x}}$ to feature points $\mathbf{x}'$.

1. Initialize parameter vector $\mathbf{b}$ to zero.
2. Generate new conditional model instance $\tilde{\mathbf{x}} = \bar{\mathbf{x}}_c + \mathbf{\Phi}\mathbf{b}$.
3. Align feature points $\mathbf{x}'$ to model $\tilde{\mathbf{x}}$.
4. Update model parameters to match the feature points, $\mathbf{b} = \mathbf{\Phi}^T(\mathbf{x}' - \bar{\mathbf{x}}_c)$.
5. Constrain $\mathbf{b}$ to be within $\pm 3\sqrt{\lambda_c}$.

6. Recover current 3D shape $\tilde{\mathbf{x}} = \bar{\mathbf{x}}_c + \boldsymbol{\Phi}\mathbf{b}$.
7. Using the current shape perform landmark displacement and iterate from Step 1.

Alignment of points is performed using Procrustes analysis [5] to eliminate rotation and translation effects. However, scale is preserved as it is an important feature in cardiac image segmentation.

3   Results

The goal of this paper is to show the potential in using commonly available patient information to construct personalized shape models that improve the accuracy of image segmentation. To test the extent of this improvement, we compare the segmentation accuracy obtained with a standard shape-only PDM to the accuracy obtained with the proposed metadata-constrained PDM. Both PDMs were trained using 150 datasets, and tested on the remaining 100 cases.

3.1   Data

Image. We used 250 cardiac magnetic resonance imaging (CMR) datasets obtained from the Cardiac Atlas Project (CAP). CAP is a web-accessible resource (www.cardiacatlas.org), comprising a population atlas of asymptomatic and pathological hearts [4]. For this study we use 250 asymptomatic cases from the Multi Ethnic Study of Atherosclerosis (MESA) study [1]. The MESA protocol used fast gradient-recalled echo (GRE) imaging with 10–12 short axis slices with typical parameters 6 mm thickness, 4 mm gap, field of view 360–400 mm, 256×160 matrix, and pixel size from 1.4–2.5 mm/pixel depending on patient size.

Shape. Contours were manually drawn as a series of points by the MESA CMR core lab on short-axis slices for all cases at end-diastole (ED). These contours were fitted by a finite element model by linear least squares as described in [7]. The resulting models are 250 triangular meshes with point correspondence. The meshes are comprised of 1570 points, of which 785 describe the endocardial surface at ED. In this paper we focus on the shape analysis of the Left Ventricular (LV) endocardial surface at ED.

Metadata. In this study we include the following metadata fields provided along with the image data: age, gender, race, height, weight, systolic/diastolic blood pressure, heart rate, hypertension, smoker, alcohol. Some of these fields are continuous variables and others are categorical. All categorical variables were replaced by binary codes of length n, where n is the number of categories for any of the variables.

3.2   Standard vs. Metadata-Constrained Segmentation

All image volumes were initialized by artificially aligning an instance of the PDM's mean shape with the ground truth. The dimension of image profiles for feature extraction was set to 7×1 voxels (3 on each side) projected inwardly and outwardly from the landmark point. The stopping criterion for the ASM was set at 30 iterations.

Table 1 shows the summary statistics for the segmentation. The root-mean-square (RMS) point-to-surface (P2S) segmentation error across all cases for the standard PDM was 2.18 mm, whereas the error for the proposed technique was 2.03 mm. This represents an accuracy improvement of 7 % over the standard PDM. Also, the standard deviation of the error was improved by 13 % over the standard PDM.

Table 1. Summary statistics comparing P2S RMS segmentation errors of the standard PDM vs. our proposed metadata-constrained PDM.

	Mean $\pm\ \sigma$ (mm)	Min.	Max.
Standard PDM	2.18 ± 0.62	1.41	4.33
Conditional PDM	2.03 ± 0.54	1.38	4.16
Improvement (%)	$7\% \pm 13\%$	-7.5%	30.4%

Figure 1 shows the percentage of improvement obtained for each individual subject plotted from lowest to highest improvement. From the figure we can see that using metadata improves the segmentation of nearly 80 % of the subjects. Additionally, in more than 20 % of subjects the segmentation accuracy was improved by a significant 15 % to 30 %.

Table 2 shows the distribution of the errors in the test sample for both the conditional- and standard-PDM segmentations. It can be seen how the use of the metadata reduces the number of cases with large errors. For example, by using the standard shape models, 59 % of the datasets are segmented with over 2 mm errors. This number is reduced to 39 % when adding the metadata during segmentation. Similarly, with the standard shape models, only 3 % of the cases are segmented with less than 1.5 mm errors, while this number increases to 14 % by using the proposed metadata constrained segmentation framework. Table 2 illustrates the positive effect of taking into account the patient metadata, in addition to shape and image information, during cardiac segmentation.

3.3   Examples

Figure 2 shows two typical examples where our technique outperforms the standard PDM. Both panels, left and right, show the segmentation obtained with the standard PDM (left), and our technique (right) superimposed on the ground truth shape. On Example 1 (left panel), the standard PDM (left) fails to correctly

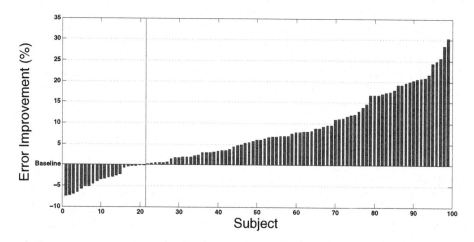

Fig. 1. Percentage of improvement provided by our metadata-constrained models. Improvements are shown in ascending order for all subjects.

Table 2. Distribution of cases by error range between the standard PDM and our proposed metadata-constrained PDM.

	Error $< x$ mm (% of Cases)			
	<1.5 mm	<2 mm	<2.5 mm	<3 mm
Standard PDM	3 %	41 %	76 %	94 %
Conditional PDM	14 %	61 %	88 %	97 %

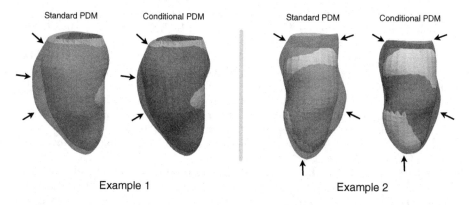

Example 1   Example 2

Fig. 2. Segmentation examples. The blue and red shapes (left and right on each example) are segmentations obtained with the standard PDM, and our conditional PDM respectively. The ground truth shape is overlaid in gray color for comparison (Color figure online).

match lateral wall of the LV, whereas our method (right) better approximates the region. Some arrows are placed on the figure to show the regions where these differences are most significant. Similarly, example 2 (right panel) shows large errors, on the basal, apical and lateral wall regions for the standard PDM (left), while our method (right) is able to match those same regions with significantly smaller errors.

4   Conclusion

We presented a method for the construction of statistical shape models that incorporate non-image information from the patient. The proposed models reduce the shape domain to custom fit the patient's unique characteristics. We achieved this by using multivariate conditional distributions to regress a model that represents the most likely shape variation given the patient's metadata. We validated our method by comparing the segmentation accuracy obtained with a standard PCA-based method with the accuracy obtained with our technique. Results showed a 7 % average segmentation improvement and in many cases improvements of up to 30 % over the standard PCA model. As future work, we would like to identify the metadata that best predicts shape and a methodology to optimally combine them such that segmentation accuracy is maximally improved.

References

1. Bild, D.E., Bluemke, D.A., Burke, G.L., Detrano, R., Roux, A.V.D., Folsom, A.R., Greenland, P., Jacobs Jr., D.R., Kronmal, R., Liu, K., et al.: Multi-ethnic study of atherosclerosis: objectives and design. Am. J. Epidemiol. **156**(9), 871–881 (2002)
2. Blanc, R., Reyes, M., Seiler, C., Székely, G.: Conditional variability of statistical shape models based on surrogate variables. In: Yang, G.-Z., Hawkes, D., Rueckert, D., Noble, A., Taylor, C. (eds.) MICCAI 2009, Part II. LNCS, vol. 5762, pp. 84–91. Springer, Heidelberg (2009)
3. Cootes, T.F., Taylor, C.J., Cooper, D.H., Graham, J.: Active shape models-their training and application. Comput. Vis. Image Understand. **61**(1), 38–59 (1995)
4. Fonseca, C.G., Backhaus, M., Bluemke, D.A., Britten, R.D., Do Chung, J., Cowan, B.R., Dinov, I.D., Finn, J.P., Hunter, P.J., Kadish, A.H., et al.: The cardiac atlas projectan imaging database for computational modeling and statistical atlases of the heart. Bioinformatics **27**(16), 2288–2295 (2011)
5. Goodall, C.: Procrustes methods in the statistical analysis of shape. J. Roy. Stat. Soc. B Stat. Meth. **53**, 285–339 (1991)
6. Grbić, S., Swee, J.K.Y., Ionasec, R.: ShapeForest: building constrained statistical shape models with decision trees. In: Fleet, D., Pajdla, T., Schiele, B., Tuytelaars, T. (eds.) ECCV 2014, Part III. LNCS, vol. 8691, pp. 597–612. Springer, Heidelberg (2014)
7. Medrano-Gracia, P., Cowan, B.R., Ambale-Venkatesh, B., Bluemke, D.A., Eng, J., Finn, J.P., Fonseca, C.G., Lima, J.A., Suinesiaputra, A., Young, A.A.: Left ventricular shape variation in asymptomatic populations: the multi-ethnic study of atherosclerosis. Cardiovasc. Res. **16**(1), 56 (2014)

8. Pereanez, M., Lekadir, K., Castro-Mateos, I., Pozo, J., Lazary, A., Frangi, A.: Accurate segmentation of vertebral bodies and processes using statistical shape decomposition and conditional models. IEEE Trans. Med. Imaging **34**(8), 1627–1639 (2015)
9. Van Assen, H.C., Danilouchkine, M.G., Frangi, A.F., Ordás, S., Westenberg, J.J., Reiber, J.H., Lelieveldt, B.P.: Spasm: a 3D-ASM for segmentation of sparse and arbitrarily oriented cardiac MRI data. Med. Image Anal. **10**(2), 286–303 (2006)
10. Wolz, R., Aljabar, P., Hajnal, J.V., Lötjönen, J., Rueckert, D., Initiative, A.D.N., et al.: Nonlinear dimensionality reduction combining MR imaging with non-imaging information. Med. Image Anal. **16**(4), 819–830 (2012)

Myocardial Infarct Localization Using Neighbourhood Approximation Forests

Héloïse Bleton$^{(\boxtimes)}$, Jàn Margeta, Hervé Lombaert, Hervé Delingette,
and Nicholas Ayache

Asclepios Team, INRIA Sophia-Antipolis, Valbonne, France
bletonheloise@gmail.com

Abstract. This paper presents a machine-learning algorithm for the automatic localization of myocardial infarct in the left ventricle. Our method constructs neighbourhood approximation forests, which are trained with previously diagnosed 4D cardiac sequences. We introduce a new set of features that simultaneously exploit information from the shape and motion of the myocardial wall along the cardiac cycle. More precisely, characteristics are extracted from a hyper surface that represents the profile of the myocardial thickness. The method has been tested on a database of 65 cardiac MRI images in order to retrieve the diagnosed infarct area. The results demonstrate the effectiveness of the NAF in predicting the left ventricular infarct location in 7 distinct regions. We evaluated our method by verifying the database ground truth. Following a new examination of the 4D cardiac images, our algorithm may detect misclassified infarct locations in the database.

Keywords: Machine learning · Neighbourhood approximation forests · Myocardial infarction · Wall thickness

1 Introduction

Cardiac imaging is now routinely used for evaluating specific anatomical and functional characteristics of hearts. For instance, the localization of cardiac infarcts requires contrast agent injection and a thorough examination of the myocardial wall thickness and its motion [3,4]. We propose to assist and automate this process with a system that automatically categorizes the localization of infarcts in the left ventricle. We exploit information from existing databases of 4D cardiac image sequences, that already contain the infarct localization from previously diagnosed patients. In such context, 4D images should be compared in an image reference space.

One way to represent the population is with statistical anatomical atlases [2] that are constructed by combining all available subjects in a single average reference. In this paper, we favor a representation that considers all available subjects in a database. Here, we consider data that is classified along their recorded infarct localization. For this purpose, multi-atlas methods [5] could be used.

© Springer International Publishing Switzerland 2016
O. Camara et al. (Eds.): STACOM 2015, LNCS 9534, pp. 108–116, 2016.
DOI: 10.1007/978-3-319-28712-6_12

However, they require costly image registrations [6]. Retrieval systems, instead, find images of subjects in a database that are close to a query image [7]. The information on the infarct location of the retrieved subjects may be relevant for establishing diagnoses in previously unseen subjects.

Content based retrieval systems require the notion of distances between images [10]. They have been used in other areas such as neuro-images [11] or endomicroscopy [8]. However, to the best of our knowledge, they were not applied for categorizing infarct locations in 4D cardiac images. This raises the question on how distances between 4D images should be defined. We suggest to learn this metric between subjects that belong to different categories of infarct locations, using the Neighborhood Approximation Forests algorithm (NAF) [11]. This machine-learning approach approximates distances between new query images and images in a database, via an affinity matrix between subjects. Decision forests have already been applied for processing medical images such as a fully automatic segmentation of the left ventricle [9]. Our method builds upon simple shape and motion features derived from binary segmentation that are fast to compute and based on a hyper surface representing the myocardial thickness along the cardiac cycle.

The contribution of this paper is the use of a distance learning approach for automatically categorizing the location of cardiac infarcts from 4D cardiac image sequences. We tested several features that are extracted from a novel hyper surface representation of the thickness profile. The next section describes our localization method, and is followed by our results that evaluates the performance of the proposed features. We discuss on the differences found in our results and elaborate on future improvements of our infarct localization method.

2   Method

Our localization method consists of categorizing automatically the location of cardiac infarcts via a retrieval approach based on the Neighborhood Approximation Forests (NAF). We now suggest feature representations that are specific for the localization of infarcts in 4D cardiac image sequences. The underlying assumption is that infarction affects the myocardial shape and motion since complex phenomena are often involved, such as wall thickening or chamber dilation [3].

2.1   Neighbourhood Approximation Forests

The NAF consists of an ensemble of binary decision trees designed for the purpose of clustering similar cardiac sequences together. Its automatic learning of image neighborhoods provides the capability of querying a training dataset of images, $\mathbf{I}$, by retrieving the most similar images given a previously unseen image, J. Further details of the algorithm are described in [11]. Three phases are required: feature extraction, training and testing stages. We now describe how to apply them for the specific problem of locating infarcts in 4D images.

The learning process aims at finding the optimal shape and motion features for predicting the category of infarct location. Our training dataset contains 4D cardiac image sequences, each labeled with a category of infarct location, e.g., infarct is in septal or lateral area. Each 4D image should have an associated 4D segmentation mask of the left ventricular muscle. In our case, each binary mask has been cropped with a bounding box centered on the left ventricle and oriented such that both ventricles are aligned horizontally along a left-right axis.

Feature Extraction. A surface representing the thickness profile over the cardiac cycle is first extracted from 4D myocardial masks. The barycenter of the left ventricle mask is computed for each slice and each frame of the 4D mask. Rays are subsequently casted from the barycenter to the exterior of the mask, as illustrated on Fig. 4. The ray-binary mask intersection is used to evaluate the myocardial thickness at each angle. As a result, the myocardial thickness $h(s, t, \theta)$ is represented by a hyper surface, where the spatial coordinates are the corresponding slice s, the frame time t, and the angle θ.

The thickness profile is smoothed out by a Gaussian kernel filter (with a width of 0.4) to reduce possible segmentation errors. The thickness profile is also normalized in order to adjust its thickness values in a standardized common scale, such that the average thickness value over the 4D hyper surface is 0 and the standard deviation 1 (Fig. 1).

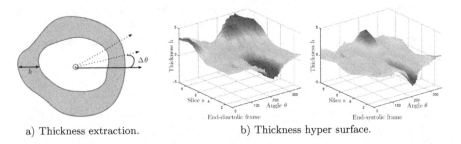

a) Thickness extraction.   b) Thickness hyper surface.

Fig. 1. (a) Thickness extraction along the myocardial mask in red, red circle shows the mask barycenter, h denotes the thickness and θ the angle of a casted ray. (b) 4D thickness profile at end-diastolic and end-systolic frames, parameterized by $h(s, t, \theta)$, with the slice s, the frame time t, and the angle θ (Color figure online).

As the space and temporal resolutions are specific to each image, point sampling should be normalized. The slice position s is normalized between 0 at the apex, and 1 at the left ventricular base. The frame time t is normalized between 0 at diastole, and 1 at the end of the cardiac cycle. The angle is kept between 0 and 2π, starting from a reference in the lateral wall.

Below, we describe groups of features $f(I)$ extracted from the thickness profiles. In the following cases, $h(s, t, \theta)$ denotes the thickness, sampled on the slice s, the frame time t and the angle θ.

Feature 1: Raw thickness. The profile constitutes the input features for each tree:

$$f_1(I) = \{h(s_i, t_j, \theta_k)\}_{i,j\in[0;1], \text{ and } \theta\in[0°;360°]}.$$

In other words, given a 4D image I, this feature representation consists of the list of surface heights. This should characterize infarcts as a function of myocardial thickness over space and time.

Feature 2: Raw thickness and thickness differences. This feature representation provides the raw thickness profile and the absolute difference of thicknesses sampled between the frame t_0 and each frame t:

$$f_2(I) = \{h(s_i, t_j, \theta_k), |h(s_i, t_0, \theta_k) - h(s_i, t_j, \theta_k)|\}_{i,j\in[0;1], \text{ and } \theta\in[0°;360°]}.$$

This feature is similar to the first feature representation, however, the thickness difference is added. This should characterize infarcts as discrepancies in myocardial thickness over space and time.

Training Phase. During this phase, the forest is trained: parameters of each tree are fixed using the training set $\mathbf{I}$ and the distance measurement $\rho(I_n, I_m)$ between each pair of images (I_n, I_m). The distance metric $\rho(I_n, I_m)$ for a regression problem is defined as follows: $\rho(I_n, I_m) = |\theta_a(I_n) - \theta_a(I_m)|$, where $\theta_a(I_n)$ denotes the angle that corresponds to the infarct location, as illustrated on Fig. 3a. A set of visual features $f(I_n)$ is computed from each training image I_n. Along the forest construction, each tree tests a randomized subset of $f(I_n)$. A tree is grown by finding at each node p, the optimal split of the dataset into two branches $(\mathbf{I}_{p_{\text{Left}}}, \mathbf{I}_{p_{\text{Right}}})$ that best separates the incoming images $\mathbf{I}_p$ in compact clusters. In the best case, cardiac images with similar infarct location should end in one leaf. In other words, the best threshold τ_p is found for each selected feature f_{m_p}. The couple (parameters m_p, threshold τ_p) are stored at each node awaiting for the testing phase.

Obtaining the most compact partioning of $\mathbf{I}_p$ is also equivalent to maximizing the information gain G (Eq. 1) at node p:

$$(m_p, \tau_p) = \arg\max_{m,\tau} G(\mathbf{I}_p, \mathbf{m}, \boldsymbol{\tau}), \tag{1}$$

where $\mathbf{m}$ is the set of features, and $\boldsymbol{\tau}$ the set of potential thresholds, and

$$G(\mathbf{I}_p, m_p, \tau_p) = C(\mathbf{I}_p) - \frac{|\mathbf{I}_{p_{\text{Right}}}|}{|\mathbf{I}_p|}C(\mathbf{I}_{p_{\text{Right}}}) - \frac{|\mathbf{I}_{p_{\text{Left}}}|}{|\mathbf{I}_p|}C(\mathbf{I}_{p_{\text{Left}}}), \tag{2}$$

where the set of images $\mathbf{I}_{p_{\text{Left}}}$ of the left child node is defined by the test function $\Gamma(m_p, \tau_p)$ applied on the images of the parent node, and similarly for the definition of the right node. Moreover, the compactness is defined by $C(A) = \frac{1}{|A|^2}\sum_{I_i\in A}\sum_{I_j\in A}\rho(I_i, I_j)$, and $|A|$ is the number of images within a subset A. More details on the training phase of the NAFs can be found in [11].

Testing Phase. During the following phase, one testing cardiac image travels across all tree nodes using the trained decisions, starting from the root node and ending in one leaf. Each leaf contains the training images for which similar decisions were taken. Consequently, when a testing image reaches a final leaf, it is considered a neighbor of the training images already present in the same final leaf. An affinity matrix is built by repeating this neighborhood approximation for each tree by storing the affinities between all testing images and the training images, as illustrated in Fig. 2.

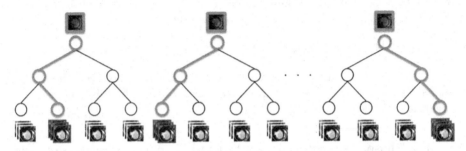

Fig. 2. The NAF testing phase. The trained NAF determines the most similar images (in the bottom/in red) of the testing cardiac sample (in the top of each tree/in green), by performing trained tests at each node (Color figure online).

Indeed, the NAF algorithm keeps a record of the most similar cardiac sequences to a testing image J_j in a similarity matrix W, where rows correspond to training images, and columns to testing images. For each tree, $W(i,j)$ is incremented when J_j reaches the leaf node that also includes the training image I_i [11]. In this paper, the resulting affinity matrix determine the angle, where the myocardial infarct is approximatively located (refer to Fig. 3). The predicted angle on a testing image J_j, is based on the resulting similarity matrix such that: $\theta_a(J_j) = \frac{\sum_i W(i,j)\theta_a(I_i)}{\sum_i W(i,j)}$.

3   Results

3.1   Dataset and Settings

Cardiac images of patients with coronary artery disease and a left ventricle infarction were randomly selected from the Defibrillators to Reduce Risk by Magnetic Resonance Imaging Evaluation database (DETERMINE) included in the Cardiac Atlas Project (CAP) [1]. 65 4D left ventricular masks were obtained with the software CAP Client, made available by the Left Ventricular Segmentation Challenge conducted for the Statistical Atlases and Computational Models of the Heart Workshop (STACOM) in 2011. Each mask is annotated by additional clinical information including the infarct location (anterior-septal, anterior, anterior-lateral, lateral, inferior-lateral, inferior, inferior-septal).

3.2   Evaluation of Infarct Localization

We validated our approach by retrieving the neighbours and the predicted angle by forming a training set and a testing set from the expert-annotated database. Some of the cardiac images are duplicated to obtain balanced class distribution in the training set. Therefore, the database consists of 115 images that groups 7 types of infarct location together.

The 10-fold cross validation technique is used for estimating the accurate performance of our classifier. The set of 115 images is partitioned into 10 subsets: 1 subset is randomly chosen as the testing set while the 9 remaining subsets form the training set. This method is repeated 10 times by varying the testing subset. Each infarct location in the dataset is labeled by an angle according to Fig. 3a. Left-ventricular regions cover large areas, spanning up to 60°. Following the testing phase of the NAF method, the predicted angle of each testing image is compared to the expected angle of infarction.

We proposed two types of features to locate the infarct of unseen cardiac images. Our forest is composed of 100 trees where the maximal depth is 20. Results associated with each type of features are shown in Fig. 3b, where the average angle of each category is reported.

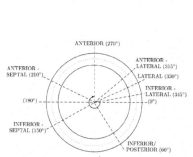

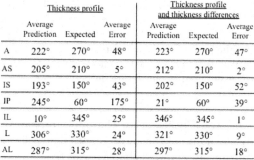

	Thickness profile			Thickness profile and thickness differences		
	Average Prediction	Expected	Average Error	Average Prediction	Expected	Average Error
A	222°	270°	48°	223°	270°	47°
AS	205°	210°	5°	212°	210°	2°
IS	193°	150°	43°	202°	150°	52°
IP	245°	60°	175°	21°	60°	39°
IL	10°	345°	25°	346°	345°	1°
L	306°	330°	24°	321°	330°	9°
AL	287°	315°	28°	297°	315°	18°

a) Sections of the left ventricular wall [12].

b) Results on average prediction of infarct location.

Fig. 3. (a) Sections of the myocardial wall related to an angle, ranging from 0° to 360°. (b) Results and comparison with the expected angle for each category: anterior (A), anterior-septal (AS), inferior-septal (IS), inferior-posterior (IP), inferior-lateral (IL), lateral (L), anterior-lateral (AL).

With the first type of features, which characterizes the thickness of the myocardium, the localization of seven areas lead to average angular errors between 5° and 48°, which are below the maximal span of each areas of 60°. However, the inferior-posterior area lead to an average error of 175°.

This leads us to examine each 4D image labeled with inferior-posterior infarct, revealing potentially misclassified infarct location, as seen on Fig. 4. The main drawback of this first type of features is that only the myocardial wall shape is taken into account, notably, only the wall thinning in the infarct area

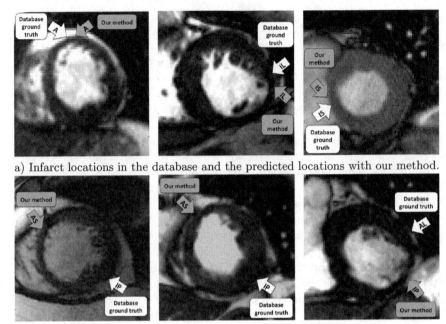

a) Infarct locations in the database and the predicted locations with our method.

b) Misclassified infarct locations in the database.

Fig. 4. The white arrows represent the database ground truth, whereas the red arrows show the infarct location that was predicted with our method. In Fig. 4b, our algorithm underlined a possible misclassification as the infarct seems located in another myocardial area (Color figure online).

or the wall thickening in the opposite wall of the infarct. Indeed, considering only the minimal thickness is not enough to localize an infarct, as the thickness of the myocardial wall changes over time and possibly gets thinner at end-systole than in the infarct area.

Motivated by the previous results, motion information is combined to shape information in the features 2 by considering the difference of thicknesses over time. Following a myocardial infarction, the cardiac wall may not necessarily change over the cardiac cycle whereas the wall thickness of a healthy heart changes over time. Consequently, our second feature type that captures the thickness differences over time infarcts should indicate infarct as areas where the thickness is not changing over time.

With the second type of features, the infarct location is predicted with an average angular error of up to 52° from the expected angle in all categories. This remains below the maximal span of each areas of 60°. Our algorithm is able to locate the infarct location within the right area even if there are potential sources of error in the dataset. For instance, the database ground truth may be corrupted by misaligned binary masks if the septum is not perfectly located at 180° as illustrated on Fig. 3a.

4   Conclusion

We used our machine learning neighbourhood-based algorithm for detecting the infarct in the left ventricular wall. We propose 2 types of features for improving the infarct localization where shape and motion information have been taken into consideration. These features have been extracted from a hyper surface that represents the thickness profile and has been designed along the cardiac cycle. We learnt to approximatively locate the infarct by retrieving the corresponding angle from the undiagnosed images. The most relevant infarct location is based on an affinity matrix. Our approach may be relevant in assisting clinical diagnosis of left ventricular infarct and may sometimes detect misclassified infarct in a database. Future work will focus on evaluating local wall deformation fields to better localize the infarct over the 3D cardiac volume. We could also consider to collect the myocardial thickness from 4D cardiac images instead of binary masks.

Acknowledgements. The authors wish to thank Alistair Young for providing the DETERMINE database. This research is partially funded by the ERC Advanced Grant MedYMAFunding.

References

1. Fonseca, C., Backhaus, M., Bluemke, D., Britten, R., Chung, J., Cowan, B., Dinov, I., Finn, J., Hunter, P., Kadish, A., Lee, D., Lima, J., Medrano-Gracia, P., Shivkumar, K., Suinesiaputra, A., Tao, W., Young, A.: The cardiac atlas project. An imaging database for computational modeling and statistical atlases of the heart. Bioinformatics **27**(16), 2288–2295 (2011)
2. Perperidis, D., Mohiaddin, R.H., Rueckert, D.: Construction of a 4D statistical atlas of the cardiac anatomy and its use in classification. In: Duncan, J.S., Gerig, G. (eds.) MICCAI 2005. LNCS, vol. 3750, pp. 402–410. Springer, Heidelberg (2005)
3. Medrano-Gracia, P., Suinesiaputra, A., Cowan, B., Bluemke, D., Frangi, A., Lee, D., Lima, J., Young, A.: An atlas for cardiac MRI regional wall motion and infarct scoring. In: Camara, O., Mansi, T., Pop, M., Rhode, K., Sermesant, M., Young, A. (eds.) STACOM 2012. LNCS, vol. 7746, pp. 188–197. Springer, Heidelberg (2013)
4. Wei, D., Sun, Y., Ong, S., Chai, P., Teo, L., Low, A.: Three-dimensional segmentation of the left ventricle in late gadolinium enhanced MR images of chronic infarction combining long-and short-axis information. Med. Image Anal. **17**(6), 685–697 (2013)
5. Rohlfing, T., Brandt, R., Menzel, R., Russakoff, D.B., Maurer Jr., C.R.: Quo vadis, atlas-based segmentation. In: Handbook of Biomedical Image Analysis, pp. 435–486. Springer US, New York (2005)
6. Heckemann, R., Keihaninejad, S., Aljabar, P., Rueckert, D., Hajnal, J., Hammers, A.: Improving intersubject image registration using tissue-class information benefits robustness and accuracy of multi-atlas based anatomical segmentation. Neuroimage **51**(1), 221–227 (2010)
7. Müller, H., Michoux, N., Bandon, D., Geissbuhler, A.: A review of content-based image retrieval systems in medical applications - clinical benefits and future directions. Int. J. Med. Inform. **73**(1), 1–23 (2004)

8. André, B., Vercauteren, T., Buchner, A., Wallace, M., Ayache, N.: A smart atlas for endomicroscopy using automated video retrieval. Med. Image Anal. **15**(4), 460–476 (2011)

9. Margeta, J., Geremia, E., Criminisi, A., Ayache, N.: Layered spatio-temporal forests for left ventricle segmentation from 4D cardiac MRI data. In: Camara, O., Konukoglu, E., Pop, M., Rhode, K., Sermesant, M., Young, A. (eds.) STACOM 2011. LNCS, vol. 7085, pp. 109–119. Springer, Heidelberg (2012)

10. Swets, D., Weng, J.: Using discriminant eigenfeatures for image retrieval. IEEE T. Pattern Anal. **8**, 831–836 (1996)

11. Konukoglu, E., Glocker, B., Zikic, D., Criminisi, A.: Neighbourhood approximation using randomized forests. Med. Image Anal. **17**(7), 790–804 (2013)

12. Cerqueira, M., Weissman, N., Dilsizian, V., Jacobs, A., Kaul, S., Laskey, W., Pennell, D., Rumberger, J., Ryan, T., Verani, M.: Standardized myocardial segmentation and nomenclature for tomographic imaging of the heart. Circulation **105**, 539–542 (2002)

Shape Challenge Papers

Systo-Diastolic LV Shape Analysis by Geometric Morphometrics and Parallel Transport Highly Discriminates Myocardial Infarction

Paolo Piras[1], Luciano Teresi[2(✉)], Stefano Gabriele[2], Antonietta Evangelista[1], Giuseppe Esposito[1], Valerio Varano[2], Concetta Torromeo[1], Paola Nardinocchi[1], and Paolo Emilio Puddu[1]

[1] Sapienza, Università di Roma, 00184 Roma, Italy
[2] Roma Tre University, 00146 Roma, Italy
teresi@uniroma3.it

Abstract. We present a procedure that detects myocardial infarction by analyzing left ventricular shapes recorded at end-diastole and end-systole, involving both shape and statistical analyses. In the framework of Geometric Morphometrics, we use Generalized Procrustes Analysis, and optionally an Euclidean Parallel Transport, followed by Principal Components Analysis to analyze the shapes. We then test the performances of different classification methods on the dataset. Among the different datasets and classification methods used, we found that the best classification performance is given by the following workflow: full shape (epicardium+endocardium) analyzed in the Shape Space (i.e. by scaling shapes at unit size); successive Parallel Transport centered toward the Grand Mean, in order to detect pure deformations; final statistical analysis via Support Vector Machine with radial basis Gaussian function. Healthy individuals show both a stronger contraction and a shape difference in systole with respect to pathological subjects. Moreover, endocardium clearly presents a larger deformation when contrasted with epicardium. Eventually, the solution for the blind test dataset is given. When using Support Vector Machine for learning from the whole training dataset and for successively classifying the 200 blind test dataset, we obtained 96 subjects classified as normal and 104 classified as pathological. After the disclosure of the blind dataset this resulted in 95 % of total accurracy with sensitivity at 97 % and specificity at 93 %.

Keywords: Geometric morphometrics · Statistical shape analysis

1 Introduction

We present a procedure able to detect myocardial infarction by analyzing Left Ventricular (LV) shapes, under the assumption that statistical shape analysis

Electronic supplementary material The online version of this chapter (doi:10.1007/978-3-319-28712-6_13) contains supplementary material, which is available to authorized users.

© Springer International Publishing Switzerland 2016
O. Camara et al. (Eds.): STACOM 2015, LNCS 9534, pp. 119–129, 2016.
DOI: 10.1007/978-3-319-28712-6_13

can predict a patient disease status. Such a procedure involves two main issues: shape analysis and statistical analysis

As regards shape analysis, Geometric Morphometrics offers the most used tool, very effective when shape data are based on homologous landmarks, i.e. Generalized Procrustes Analysis (GPA) [1,2]. GPA may be performed in both Size-and-Shape Space (SSS) or Shape Space (SS); it centers and optimally rotates shapes, optionally scaling to unit size, in order to remove non-shape informed attributes. Usually, GPA is followed by a Principal Components Analysis (PCA) performed on aligned coordinates, which gives a ranking of the main shape-change modes; PCA can be linear or non-linear, and allows visualizing main shape-change modes.

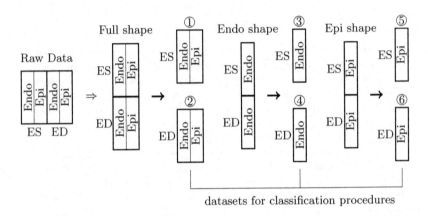

datasets for classification procedures

Fig. 1. Data handling: Given the raw data, we consider as representative of the LV configurations three different shape-data: the full shape, the endocardial shape, and the epicardial shape. On each of the three datasets, containing 800 shapes, we perform different types of shape analyses whose outcome is split in end-diastolic (ED) or end-systolic (ES) data, numbered from 1 to 6 in the Figure, and then submitted to classification procedures.

A major issue in motion sampling is the generation of homologous landmarks for each time frame, and the selection of homologous time instants along the cardiac cycle; as example, in [3] end-diastolic (ED) and end-systolic (ES) data were analyzed, in [4,5] the entire cardiac revolution was analyzed, and evaluated at homologous electro-mechanical times.

Another key issue is the discrimination among shape differences and motion differences: two left ventricles having quite different ED and ES shapes may beat in the same way, that is the deformation from ED to ES is the same. A fundamental distinction should be made in the context of shape analysis: is the between-groups shape difference the objective of the analysis or rather the deformation differences occurring between them? This question applies only if, for the same subject, at least two different shapes corresponding to two different times

Table 1. The 30 different types of shape analyses submitted to classification procedures; note that parallel transport (PT) can be centered in at least two ways, i.e. in ED or in GM. cED=centered in diastole; cGM=centered in grand mean.

Analysis Type → Dataset for classification ↓	GPA-SSS PCA	GPA-SS PCA	GPA-SSS PT - cED PCA	GPA-SS PT - cED PCA	GPA-SSS PT - cGM PCA	GPA-SS PT - cGM PCA
(1) Endo+Epi ES	1	7	13	16	19	22
(2) Endo+Epi ED	2	8	-	-	25	28
(3) Endo ES	3	9	14	17	20	23
(4) Endo ED	4	10	-	-	26	29
(5) Epi ES	5	11	15	18	21	23
(6) Epi ED	6	12	-	-	27	30

such as ED and ES, appear in the dataset [3]. Optionally, a complete sequence of shapes, representing the entire cardiac revolution, might be included in the analysis as in [4,5]. Shape differences can be gauged with standard GPA+PCA; its drawback is the mixing of inter- and intra- individual variations, thus preventing the detection of deformation patterns.

When a dataset contains many individuals, each represented by several shapes varying in time, the filtering of inter-individual differences is important. This point underlies many analytical consequences impacting the strategies aimed at exploring the shape data. In fact, while shape differences can be evaluated using standard GPA+PCA, the motion differences among groups should imply the eradication of inter-individual differences. This is necessary because, if a dataset contains different individuals, each represented by several shapes varying in time, standard GPA+PCA ineluctably mix inter- and intra- individual variations, thus preventing the appreciation of pure motion patterns. This problem can be solved by estimating deformations occurring within each individual, and by applying them to a mannequin, which can be the Grand Mean (GM) of the entire dataset, or another appropriately chosen configuration. Of course, the mannequin represents the same shape for all individuals, and in correspondence of it shape differences literally disappear, as it does not vary among individuals. In [4,5] the GM was used, thus making both ED and ES recognizable as deformed states, but another option could be that of centering in ED, depending upon the disease under study, while ES should never be erased since it contains information about inotropic state.

The geometrical tool needed for such operation is the Levi Civita Parallel Transport (PT) and the workflow of shape analysis becomes GPA+PT+PCA. It is possible to prove that once all the shapes have been optimally aligned (via GPA), an Euclidean translation can well approximate PT on the Riemannian manifold [6]. This kind of PT has the desirable property to maintain the size increment when transporting deformations in SSS (size is here defined as the square root of the summed squared distances of each landmark to the centroid).

As regards statistical analysis, classification problems are a central topic in clinical practice for a wide range of medical fields [7,8]. However, both the nature of the data and the statistical procedures used for classifying training versus test datasets make this step highly situation-specific. Recently, besides classical methods such as Linear Discriminant Analysis (LDA) and Logistic Regression (LR), several other methods entered classification practice e.g. Quadratic Discriminant Analysis (QDA), Support Vector Machine (SVM), Neural Networks (NN) and Random Forest (RF) among others, whose comparison could be challenging [9–11].

As a consequence, in any specific classification problem a comparison among different classification methods should be performed. In particular, both sensitivity and specificity should be evaluated as they have an unbalanced weight in clinics. For example, in [9] it was suggested that, while SVM shows high accuracy, its sensitivity is low with respect to other methods. In addition, a goodness of fit test, such as Hosmer Lomeshow test should be always performed in order to evaluate the distribution of predictions in deciles.

2   Methods

Raw data includes 400 left ventricles (200 for training, plus 200 blind), sampled with epi- and endo-cardial landmarks, at both ES and ED, for a total of 800 shapes, [12]. From the point of view of shape analysis, ES and ED must be regarded as different shapes; thus, we organize our dataset as a list of 800 shapes, and we consider three sub shape-data: (1) full shapes, consisting of both epicardial and endocardial data; (2) endocardial shapes; (3) epicardial shapes, see Fig. 1. We apply both the GPA+PCA and GPA+PT+PCA strategies to the three aforementioned shape-data, in both SSS and SS, and using PT with two different data centering (i.e. in the Grand Mean or in Diastole), thus totalling 30 different sub-analyses which provide the PC scores to be used for classification procedures, see Table 1; it is worth noting that all 800 shapes have to undergo a common GPA+PCA or GPA+PT+PCA; once shape analysis has been done, the 800 PC scores are split in ED or ES data, each with 400 cases: these will be the datasets to be used for classification procedures.

We use five classification procedures: LDA, LR, QDA, RF and SVM with Gaussian Radial Basis Kernel Function. To assess the performances of the five different procedures, we use only the labelled training dataset, that is, half of the 400 cases (100 healthy + 100 pathological) as follows:

1. At first, using the whole training dataset, and for any of the 30 types of shape analyses, we perform an univariate association filtering via ANOVA on the first 100 PC scores. The design is a classical one-way ANOVA using the training affiliation healthy/pathological as a two-levels factor. P-value was set (conservatively) to 0.05. All significant PC scores are retained for classifications.
2. We assemble a *warm-up dataset* by randomly extracting 50 healthy individuals, and 50 patients affected by Myocardial Infarction (MI) from the training

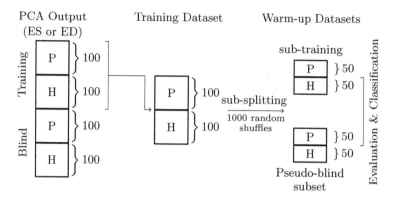

Fig. 2. Once shape analysis has been done on the whole shape-dataset, only the training subset is considered for classification method selection; from the training subset we assemble a learning dataset, composed of a sub-train and a sub-test dataset (not blind), by randomly selecting 50 healthy and 50 pathological cases to fill each of the two sub-datasets. The assembly is repeated and analyzed 1000 times. ES=end-systolic data, ED=end-diastolic data, P=Pathology, H=Healthy.

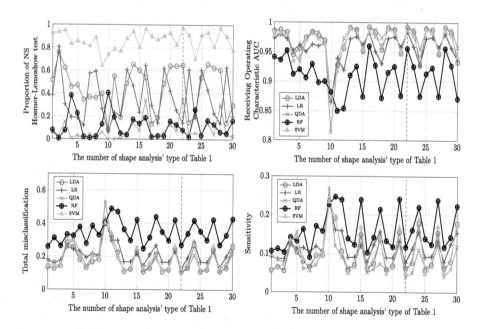

Fig. 3. Top left: Proportion of non significant H-L test over the 1000 classification simulations performed for the 5 methods on any type of shape analysis. Ordinal positions on x-axis correspond to shape analysis' types in Table 1. Top right: Corresponding mean AUC over 1000 simulations. Best performances, in all panels, according to H-L test and ROC AUC is for type 22 (vertical, dashed line). Bottom left: Mean total misclassification over 1000 simulations. Bottom right: Mean sensitivity over 1000 simulations.

Table 2. We report the scores for the 30 types of analyses resulting from SVM; they show the higher percentage of non significant H-L test in comparison to other classification methods. Figures represent SVM proportions and AUC as in Fig. 3.

Type of analysis	1	2	3	4	5	6	7	8	9	10	11	12	13	14	15
Non Sig. H-L test	0.93	0.94	0.95	0.83	0.86	0.84	0.81	0.89	0.64	0.74	0.79	0.77	0.88	0.94	0.80
Total misclass	0.15	0.14	0.15	0.30	0.29	0.19	0.13	0.20	0.19	0.40	0.34	0.22	0.11	0.13	0.25
Sensitivity	0.06	0.06	0.07	0.13	0.14	0.09	0.06	0.10	0.10	0.23	0.19	0.10	0.05	0.06	0.17
AUC	0.98	0.98	0.98	0.93	0.94	0.97	0.98	0.97	0.96	0.87	0.92	0.96	0.99	0.98	0.95
Type of analysis	16	17	18	19	20	21	22	23	24	25	26	27	28	29	30
Non Sig. H-L test	0.96	0.90	0.87	0.90	0.93	0.83	0.97	0.91	0.70	0.91	0.93	0.81	0.97	0.90	0.78
Total misclass	0.13	0.16	0.21	0.11	0.13	0.26	0.13	0.16	0.27	0.11	0.13	0.27	0.13	0.16	0.26
Sensitivity	0.06	0.08	0.14	0.05	0.06	0.17	0.05	0.08	0.19	0.05	0.07	0.17	0.05	0.09	0.17
AUC	0.98	0.98	0.96	0.99	0.98	0.95	0.99	0.98	0.94	0.99	0.98	0.95	0.99	0.98	0.94

dataset; this procedure yields a learning training subset and a pseudo-blind subset, each containing 100 cases (i.e. 50 healthy and 50 pathological), see Fig. 2.
3. We use this training subset in the 5 classification methods and we employ their learning functions in order to predict the pseudo-blind dataset; given that this is not blind, we can evaluate the performance of each classification method.

Steps (2) and (3) are repeated 1000 times. Basing on the corresponding results we counted total misclassified cases and their two components, e.g. Sensitivity and Specificity. Hosmer Lomeshow test (H-L test) was used in order to assess the Goodness of Fit of any classification problem. Receiving Operating Curves (ROC) and the Area under the Curve (AUC) were also computed. The type of shape analysis and the classification method with the best global performance in classifying the 1000 random sub-test datasets were successively used for classifying the blind test dataset. As primary criterion, we choose the percentage of non significant H-L test (the higher the better) in order to select the best classification method.

The use of H-L test as a primary criterion deserves particular attention. In fact, two classifications could have identical AUCs, sensitivities and specificities but the distributions of probabilities corresponding to misclassified cases can be very different. H-L test divides subjects into deciles based on predicted probabilities, then computes a chi-square from observed and expected frequencies. For example, in two different classifications, the probabilities of misclassified cases can be around 0.5. Or they can have values (leading to wrong classification) close to 0 or 1. In the latter case the severity of misclassification is worse.

Only for the best type analysis selected with this method, we also re-run a non linear PCA based on the Relative Warps Analysis (RWA) [2]. RWA uses the Thin Plate Spline (TPS) interpolation function in order to compute and visualize the deformation occurring between a reference and a target shape. RWA, with the associated scores, yields a sequence of ordered subspaces onto which each

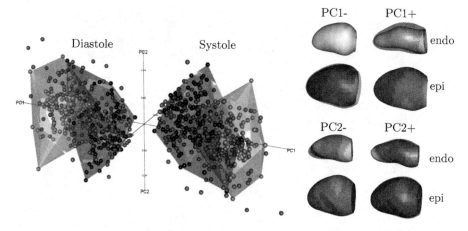

Fig. 4. PCA results for type of analysis 22. Left: Shapes in the PC1-PC3 space; green=healthy, black=MI, red=blind. Right: 3D shape corresponding to PC1 and PC2 modes, colored according to the distance with respect to the GM (blue: minimum; red: maximum) (Color figure online).

single case is projected. Warping is parametrized by the α parameter: for $\alpha = 1$, large-scale variations (variations among specimens in the relative positions of widely separated landmarks) are given more weight with respect to the small-scale ones; for $\alpha = -1$, the opposite is true, and more weight is given to variation in the relative positions of landmarks that are close together. A value of $\alpha = 0$ yields to virtually identical results of a linear PCA on Procrustes coordinates. More details can be found in [13,14]. To detect the importance of large- or small-scale variations, the exponent α of the bending energy matrix was set equal to 1, 0 (corresponding to standard PCA), and -1. On the resulting RW scores of these three types of RWA we run the best classification method found when using standard PCA. The results were compared with the standard PCA results and the absolute best result is used for classifying the blind dataset.

3   Results

In Fig. 3 results of performances of the five methods are shown. It appears evident that SVM with Gaussian Radial Basis kernel function is characterized, under the 1000 simulations, by a higher probability to present a non significant H-L test. Table 2 reports the results relative to the 30 types of analyses (only for SVM) that shows the higher percentage of non significant H-L test in comparison to other methods. Analysis type 22 is the best for H-L evaluation; it uses the full shape for shape analysis, subjected to a GPA-SS, plus PT-cGM (PT centered in Grand Mean), plus PCA; then, only systolic data are used for statistical analysis.

Among the firsts 100 PC scores for analysis type 22, the univariate association filtering found 1, 2, 3, 5, 6, 8, 12, 13, 21, 24, 31, 38, 57, significant (significance

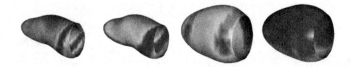

Fig. 5. From left to right: endocardium for healthy; endocardium for pathological; epicardium for healthy; epicardium for pathological. Color denotes the distance with respect to the GM (blue: minimum; red: maximum) (Color figure online).

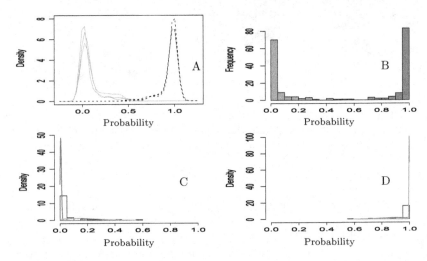

Fig. 6. A: probability-density distributions emerging from our classification of the blind dataset. Only the results obtained with the optimal analysis method (type 22) and the first two sub-optimal ones (types 16 and 28) are presented. B: the corresponding histograms. C: healthy-subject distribution fitted by the sum of two normal distributions. D: pathological-subject distribution fitted by the sum of two normal distributions.

level $= 0.05$) by using the known healthy/pathological affiliation as binary factor. These PC scores were used to select the best classification method.

We found that, in comparison to results of Table 2, RWA performed on the type of analysis 22 with $\alpha = -1$ yields a lowest percentage of misclassification (8 %), and of significant H-L test (1.9 %) after re-running the resampling procedure we described above. RW scores significant in the univariate association filtering were: 1~5, 7~10, 15, 16, 20, 38, 74. Moreover, mean AUC was slightly improved (99.3), the sensitivity reduced (3 %), as well as total misclassification (8 %). RWA on type of analysis 22 with $\alpha = -1$ will then be used in order to predict the blind test dataset.

Figure 4 (left) shows the 800 shapes in PCA scatterplot corresponding to the type of analysis 22. Healthy individuals (green) clearly set apart from pathological ones (black), while blind (red) subjects are dispersed across the two distributions; see also Supplementary Figure S1 with dynamic 3D pdf (requires Adobe Reader).

Deformations associated to PC1 and PC2 extremes are also shown in Fig. 4: we plot the values of $\|x_M - x\|$, with x_M the position of a point in the GM, and x its position at ED or ES; the colormap ranges from blue (min) to red (max). It is evident that PC1 represents contraction. This contraction is more evident on the endocardium than in epicardium and healthy individuals occupy a more extreme position, along PC1, than pathological individuals. This can be better appreciated in Fig. 5 where mean deformations (relative to the Grand Mean) of healthy and pathological individuals are illustrated conjointly. Clearly healthy subjects undergo a larger, thus more efficient, contraction than MI patients even in the epicardium. The larger shape differences occur in the middle of endocardial geometry. It is important to note here that we illustrated endocardium and epicardium separately for sake of clarity while actually in type of analysis 22 they were analyzed together as a whole geometry (thus one inside the other). See also Supplementary Figure S2.

Using SVM for learning from the whole training dataset and for successively classifying the blind test dataset, and RWA with $\alpha = -1$, we obtained 96 subjects classified as normal and 104 classified as pathological. After the disclosure of the blind dataset this resulted in 95 % of total accurracy with sensitivity at 97 % and specificity at 93 %.

We are thus able to report, case by case, the resulting classification and the probability of being found pathological according to the specified learning function. Figure 6 shows the per-class density distributions of this probability. We illustrated the results coming from type of analysis 22 (our optimal result) together with the first two sub-optimal types, i.e. types 16 and 28. The two curves are pretty similar and the 0/1 classifications are much similar among the three types. It is evident that the two groups are well separated with very few cases possessing probabilities around 0.5.

The distributions of the two probabilities suggest that, within each class, more than one normal distribution is represented. This could be evidence of a few pre-clinical healthy individuals and a few only moderately pathological subjects.

The fact that RWA with $\alpha = -1$ performs better in discriminating healthy from pathological subjects could be related to physiological evidences: myocardial infarction is a particularly localized pathology. It can be transmural or subendocardial, but in both cases a relatively small region of LV is interested. This region can be found at several LV locations, and $\alpha = -1$ gives more importance to small scale variations; this is coherent with this particular type of pathology. On the opposite, for example, a pathology that moulds the entire LV shape, such as Aortic Regurgitation could be better discriminated using $\alpha = 1$. Testing this is beyond the scope of the present paper.

However, this result suggests that a tuned evaluation of deformation could correlate with the deep nature of pathology. Another result that should be commented is the evidence that the full shape (i.e. epicardium+endocardium) better discriminates than epicardium or endocardium alone. Given that the location of infarction was not known for the available sample of pathological individuals, we can only speculate that the lesser contraction of pathological condition evidenced in Fig. 5 is inevitably related to a lesser extent of myocardial thickness variation and that this feature can only be recognized by analyzing together epicardium and endocardium.

Finally, it has also to be pointed out that the relative age of infarction, whose information was missing in the blind dataset, might be a further factor contributing to diagnostic accuracy. It is in fact well known that LV undergoes a time-dependent overall shape change post-infarction which was variably interpreted and measured but is in general termed "remodeling", just to underscore that not only the infarcted area but also the remaining still healthy LVs undergo modifications to adapt, globally, to the loss of viable contracting muscle. As remodeling might be minimal in some cases due to a little recent infarction or to a relatively old one and stabilized, the double normal distributions seen in Fig. 6 (pathological side) might represent these conditions. On the other hand, subclinical and localized ischemia might, on the "healthy" side, explain the double distribution there. Clearly, these are speculations and only the full disclosure of the blind database will enable adequate considerations.

4   Conclusions

Deformation analysis performs better than shape analysis alone in detecting pathology. This can be done by adding the PT to standard GPA+PCA. This allows recovering the attributes linked to the contraction process *per-se* that, ultimately, follows the mechanics of heart functioning. Filtering inter-individual shape differences becomes, thus, very important when exploring systo-diastolic shape changes occurring in a blind sample of healthy subjects and patients affected by Myocardial Infarction.

References

1. Adams, D.C., Rohlf, F.J., Slice, D.E.: Geometric morphometrics: ten years of progress following the revolution. Ital. J. Zool. **71**, 5–16 (2004)
2. Dryden, I.L., Mardia, K.V.: Statistical Shape Analysis. Wiley, Chichester (1998)
3. Zhang, X., Cowan, B.R., Bluemke, D.A., Finn, J.P., Fonseca, C.G., Kadish, A.H., Lee, D.C., Lima, J.A.C., Suinesiaputra, A., Young, A.A., Medrano-Gracia, P.: Atlas-based quantification of cardiac remodeling due to myocardial infarction. PLoS ONE **9**(10), e110243 (2014)
4. Piras, P., Evangelista, A., Gabriele, S., Nardinocchi, P., Teresi, L., Torromeo, C., Schiariti, M., Varano, V., Puddu, P.E.: 4D-analysis of left ventricular heart cycle using Procrustes motion analysis. Plos One **9**, e86896 (2014)
5. Madeo, A., Piras, P., Re, F., Gabriele, S., Nardinocchi, P., Teresi, L., Torromeo, C., Chialastri, C., Schiariti, M., Giura, G., Evangelista, A., Dominici, T., Varano, V., Zachara, E., Puddu, P.E.: A new 4D trajectory-based approach unveils abnormal LV revolution dynamics in hypertrophic cardiomyopathy. PloS One **10**(4), e0122376 (2015)

6. Varano, V., Gabriele, S., Teresi, L., Dryden, I., Puddu, P.E., Torromeo, C., Piras, P.: Comparing shape trajectories of biological soft tissues in the size-and-shape. BIOMAT 2014 Congress Book (in press, 2015)

7. Efron, B.: The efficiency of logistic regression compared to normal discriminant analysis. J. Am. Stat. Assoc. **70**, 892–898 (1975)

8. Peter, C.A.: A comparison of regression trees, logistic regression, generalized additive models, and multivariate adaptive regression splines for predicting AMI mortality. Stat. Med. **26**, 2937–2957 (2007)

9. Maroco, J., Silva, D., Rodrigues, A., Guerreiro, M., Santana, I., de Mendonça, A.: Data mining methods in the prediction of Dementia: a real-data comparison of the accuracy, sensitivity and specificity of linear discriminant analysis, logistic regression, neural networks, support vector machines, classification trees and random forests. BMC Res. Notes **4**, 299 (2011)

10. Puddu, P.E., Menotti, A.: Artificial neural networks versus proportional hazards Cox models to predict 45-year all-cause mortality in the Italian Rural Areas of the Seven Countries Study. BMC Res. Methodol. **12**, 100 (2011)

11. Goss, E.P., Ramchandani, H.: Comparing classification accuracy of neural networks, binary logit regression and discriminant analysis for insolvency prediction of life insurers. J. Econ. Finan. **19**, 1–18 (1995)

12. Fonseca, C.G., Backhaus, M., Bluemke, D.A., Britten, R.D., Do Chung, J., Cowan, B.R., Dinov, I.D., Finn, J.P., Hunter, P.J., Kadish, A.H., Lee, D.C., Lima, J.A.C., Medrano-Gracia, P., Shivkumar, K., Suinesiaputra, A., Tao, W., Young, A.A.: The cardiac atlas project: an imaging database for computational modeling and statistical atlases of the heart. Bioinformatics **27**(16), 2288–2295 (2011)

13. Bookstein, F.L.: Morphometric Tools for Landmark Data. Cambridge University Press, Cambridge (1991)

14. Rohlf, F.J.: Relative warp analysis and an example of its application to mosquito wings. In: Marcus L.F., Bello E., García-Valdecasa A., (eds.) Contributions to morphometrics, Museu Nacionale de Ciencias Naturales, pp. 131–159 (1993)

Statistical Shape Modeling Using Partial Least Squares: Application to the Assessment of Myocardial Infarction

Karim Lekadir[1]([✉]), Xènia Albà[1], Marco Pereañez[1], and Alejandro F. Frangi[2]

[1] Center for Computational Imaging and Simulation Technologies in Biomedicine, Universitat Pompeu Fabra, Barcelona, Spain
karim.lekadir@upf.edu
[2] Center for Computational Imaging and Simulation Technologies in Biomedicine, University of Sheffield, Sheffield, UK

Abstract. Statistical shape modeling (SSM) is a widely popular framework in cardiac image analysis, especially for image segmentation and computer-aided diagnosis. However, the conventional PCA-based models produce new axes of variation which are statistically motivated but thus are not necessarily clinically meaningful. In this paper, we propose an alternative method for statistical decomposition of the shape variability based on partial least squares (PLS). With this method, the model construction is achieved such that it is constrained by the specific clinical question of interest (*e.g.*, estimation of disease state). To achieve this, instead of deriving modes of variation in the directions of maximal variation as in PCA, PLS searches for new axes of variation that correlate most with some output clinical response variables such as diagnostic labels, leading to a decomposition that is anatomically and clinically more meaningful. The validation carried out with 200 cases from the Cardiac Atlas Project database as part of the MICCAI 2015 challenge on SSM, including healthy and infarcted left ventricles, shows the strength of the proposed PLS-based statistical shape model, with 98 % prediction accuracy.

1 Introduction

Statistical shape modeling (SSM) is a powerful tool for the robust processing and interpretation of cardiac images. The fundamental idea is to extract from a training population a representation of the variability between individuals or within a class of disease. Most commonly, this is achieved through principal component analysis (PCA), which extracts an average cardiac shape and the directions of maximal variation. In addition to the statistical decomposition using for example PCA, particular attention needs to be given to the delineation of the training images with point correspondence between the cardiac shapes, which can be obtained automatically by using nonrigid image registration [1].

There have been at least three applications of statistical shape modeling in the case of the heart. Firstly, one can use the SSMs for generating virtual populations for cardiac simulations [2]. A second application of SSMs, which is also the most common in practice, is for cardiac image segmentation. In this case, the statistical model is used to robustly guide the image search and to ensure that only valid instances of the shape are obtained.

Finally, SSMs can be used for dysfunction analysis of cardiac morphology and function, which is the subject of this paper, and which has been achieved typically by constructing models of normality from a set of healthy hearts and identifying abnormal deviations of new subjects from the statistical model. For this application, most works have used conventional PCA-based decomposition [3, 4]. Alternative approaches have been also proposed, including using sparse PCA [5], PCA with orthomax rotation [6], inter-landmark descriptors [7, 8], and independent component analysis (ICA) [9]. A major issue with these decomposition techniques is that they are statistically moti-vated, thus leading to models that are not necessarily anatomically and/or clinically meaningful.

In this paper, we propose instead a novel method for the construction of cardiac SSMs using clinically-driven shape decompositions based on partial least squares (PLS) [10]. PLS has been used extensively as a regression tool for prediction of anatomical information and clinical response in medical imaging [11–16]. In this work, we use PLS decomposition to find the modes of variation that most correlate with some clinical response variables such as disease states. More specifically, statistical models of left ventricular end-diastolic and end-systolic shapes that are discriminative of healthy and infarcted hearts are constructed, with application to myocardial infarction assessment based on 200 cases from the Cardiac Atlas Project database, as part of the MICCAI 2015 challenge on statistical shape modeling.

2   Methods

2.1   PCA Shape Decomposition

Let us denote $\mathbf{X} = (\mathbf{x}^{(1)}, \ldots, \mathbf{x}^{(N)})$ the matrix comprising the available N training shapes after shape alignment (to remove pose differences) and mean centering (after removing the mean shape $\bar{\mathbf{x}}$ from each shape). Each shape is a vector of size $3n$, where n is the total number of landmarks. In PCA, the goal is to find the new axes of variation along which there is maximal variation. For example, we want to find the first new component $\mathbf{p}_1$ (unit vector) such that:

$$\mathbf{p}_1^T \mathbf{X} \mathbf{X}^T \mathbf{p}_1 \text{ is maximized, with } \|\mathbf{p}_1\| = 1 \tag{1}$$

It can be shown that these new components can be computed as the eigenvectors of the covariance matrix of $\mathbf{X}$. With this decomposition, a new shape can be described using this generative model:

$$\mathbf{x} = \bar{\mathbf{x}} + \mathbf{Pb} \tag{2}$$

where $\mathbf{P}$ is a matrix that encapsulates t eigenvectors describing the t main directions of variation in the model, and $\mathbf{b} = (b_1, \ldots, b_t)^T$ is a vector that encapsulates the weights that control the deviation of the new subject-specific anatomical shape $\mathbf{x}$ from the mean shape $\bar{\mathbf{x}}$. Furthermore, each unit vector $\mathbf{p}_i$ is associated with an eigenvalue l_i that describes the amount of allowed variation along each axis (typically $-3\sqrt{l_i} \pounds b_i \pounds +3\sqrt{l_i}$, which correspond to about 99 % of the variability).

Note that we only describe PCA in this paper to better justify and introduce the use of PLS decomposition and that we do not use it for classification.

2.2 PLS Shape Decomposition

While PCA finds the axes of maximum variation independently of the clinical purpose of the shape model, PLS decomposition makes sure the obtained decomposition correlates with some output variable(s), which means it can be designed to be application-oriented by careful choice of the response variables. Given N training datasets, let us denote as $\mathbf{X} = (\mathbf{x}^{(1)}, \ldots, \mathbf{x}^{(N)})$ the matrix of all the input shapes after shape alignment and mean centering, and $\mathbf{Y} = (\mathbf{y}^{(1)}, \ldots, \mathbf{y}^{(N)})$ the matrix of the corresponding clinical response variables, such as for clinical diagnostic. In this paper, we will use a single diagnostic variable y to label healthy and infarcted hearts, which is equal to 0 for healthy subjects and 1 for infarcted hearts. To relate the shapes and the clinical response variables, the simplest method is to estimate a regression model such that for each new subject the unknown diagnostic variable $\hat{y}$ (healthy or infarcted heart) can be predicted with the highest possible accuracy based on the subject-specific shape $\hat{\mathbf{x}}$ as follows:

$$\hat{y} = \hat{\mathbf{x}}^T \mathbf{A} \tag{3}$$

where A is the regression matrix of the PLS model (in fact a $3n$ dimensional vector in our case, or 3n by 1 matrix), which will be defined statistically from the training matrices X and Y, such that to:

- project each shape $\mathbf{x}$ onto a new set of shape directions that are optimal for the prediction of the response y;
- remove from $\mathbf{x}$ the shape information that is irrelevant for the prediction of y; This might include shape variability that is important for the anatomical structure under investigation but which does not play a role in the specific application (for the description of myocardial infarction for example)
- eliminate noise and artifacts from the final statistical shape model.

The requirements above can be addressed in this work based on partial least square (PLS) decomposition [17]. The aim of PLS is to perform a simultaneous decomposition of X and Y such that the score vectors obtained along the new representation axes of both the input and output matrices correlate best. This will lead to optimal predictions and to maximal interdependencies between the shapes and the output variables, making the statistical shape decomposition application-oriented as defined by the clinical response variables. This type of decomposition can be obtained through the NIPALS algorithm [10]. More specifically, we wish to extract a set of t latent variables $\mathbf{C} = (\mathbf{c}_1, \ldots, \mathbf{c}_t)$ from the input training shapes $\mathbf{X}$ that correlate most with the output training response variables **Y**. In other words, we perform a simultaneous decomposition of the input and output training data as:

$$\mathbf{X} \simeq \mathbf{PC}^T \tag{4}$$

$$\mathbf{Y} \simeq \mathbf{QD}^T \tag{5}$$

such that:

$$\mathrm{cov}[\mathbf{P}^T\mathbf{X}, \ \mathbf{Q}^T\mathbf{Y}] \text{ is maximized.} \tag{6}$$

Note that $\mathbf{P} = (\mathbf{p}_1, \ldots, \mathbf{p}_t)$ are the new PLS shape components after the decomposition, while C and **D** are the new projections for the input X and Y output matrices, respectively.

To obtain the new PLS components, we wish to decompose X and **Y** simultaneously based on Eqs. (4)–(6), leading to optimal interdependencies between the input and output data. To this end, we use a procedure in which the new shape components **P** iteratively contributes to the estimations of the new output vectors **Q** and vice-versa [10]. We do this by considering one shape component $\mathbf{p}_k$ at a time (with, $k = 1, \ldots, t$ and $\mathbf{X}_1$ initialized as **X**):

(a) Initialize $\mathbf{q}_k$ with one of the columns of **Y**.
(b) Update the shape projections $\mathbf{c}_k = \mathbf{X}_k^T \mathbf{p}_k$;
     Calculate the shape component $\mathbf{p}_k = \mathbf{X}\mathbf{c}_k$, with $\|\mathbf{p}_k\| = 3$.
(c) Update output projections $\mathbf{d}_k = \mathbf{Y}^T\mathbf{q}_k$;.
     Calculate latent output variable $\mathbf{d}_k = \mathbf{Y}\mathbf{q}_k$, with $\|\mathbf{q}_k\| = 3$.
(d) Repeat (b)-(c) until no change is noticed in $\mathbf{p}_k$.
(e) Remove the contribution of $\mathbf{p}_k$ in $\mathbf{X}_k$ for next iteration: $\mathbf{X}_{k+1} = \mathbf{X}_k - \mathbf{p}_k\mathbf{p}_k^T\mathbf{X}_k$.

It can be noticed that the vector $\mathbf{c}_k$, i.e. the kth shape weights for all samples, acts as a proxy in step (b) to estimate the output variables $\mathbf{q}_k$, and vice-versa, the shape component $\mathbf{p}_k$ is used as a proxy to estimate the output projections $\mathbf{d}_k$ in step (c). These steps connect both the input and output spaces, which influence each other during decomposition, thus enforcing the derivation of correlated shape and output clinical variables (myocardial infarction score in our case). The algorithm stops when the kth shape variable does not contribute to the predictability of the clinical outputs (using cross-validation). Subsequently, with $t = k - 1$, the shape components $\mathbf{p}_1, \ldots, \mathbf{p}_t$ are retained and used in the prediction of the clinical response based on the subject-specific shapes. The remaining shape variables are ignored as they correspond to information that is not relevant to the clinical problem, or even detrimental (*e.g.*, noise or irrelevant shape variation), to the prediction of the clinical responses (e.g., disease state).

With this decomposition, the new shape components **P** are not those that maximize variation in the shape space as in PCA, but rather those that maximize co-variation with the output clinical responses, leading to models that are more clinically meaningful (see difference between the decompositions in Eqs. (1) and (6)).

2.3   Prediction of Myocardial Infarction

Based on the decomposition obtained in previous section, we obtain a shape model similar to the one generated via PCA in Eq. (2) but based on the $\mathbf{P}$ components obtained through PLS. However, these new components can also be used to predict the clinical response such as cardiac disease state based on the regression model introduced in Eq. (3). More specifically, it can be shown that for a new shape $\hat{\mathbf{x}}$, its disease state can be estimated by using in Eq. (3) the following regression matrix:

$$\mathbf{A} = \mathbf{XD}(\mathbf{P}^T\mathbf{XX}^T\mathbf{Q})^{-1}\mathbf{P}^T\mathbf{Y}. \tag{7}$$

It is important to note that for our myocardial infarction application, the response variable y is categorical (0 for healthy subjects and 1 for cases with myocardial infarction). Yet, the PLS prediction in Eq. (7) outputs a continuous response scalar, which we transform into a categorical value for the discrimination between healthy and infarcted hearts as follows:

$$y = \begin{cases} 0 \text{ (healthy subject)} & \text{if } y < 0.5 \\ 1 \text{ (infarcted heart)} & \text{if } y > 0.5. \end{cases} \tag{8}$$

Alternatively, one could also consider the PLS discriminant analysis technique, which can directly model categorical variables [18, 19].

2.4   Fusion of PLS Classifiers

Fusion of classifiers is a common approach to increase the classification accuracy in medical image compution. The idea is to combine the results from different classifiers as obtained for example by using different parameters tunings or algorithm properties. This is generally done probabilistically, *i.e.* by chosing the classification which max-imal agreement amongst the different classifiers. In our case, different different PLS classifiers of myocardial infarction can be obtained by using varying numbers of latent variables. To fuse these distinct classifications, we simply propose to use an odd number K of PLS classifiers by using the numbers of latents variables $t_1, \ldots, t_K$ and to subsequently derive a final classification by combining the muliple PLS classifications $y_1, \ldots, y_K$ using a simple medican approach as follow:

$$y = \underset{i=1,\ldots K}{\text{median}}(y_i). \tag{9}$$

The K PLS classifiers to be used as input for the fusion should be chosen empir-ically at training, *i.e.* by selecting a set of numbers of latent variables that produce the best responses in cross-validation tests as illustrated in the result section (see Sect. 3.2).

3   Results

3.1   Datasets

The proposed technique is validated in the context of the MICCAI 2015 Statistical Shape Modeling challenge (SSM2015). The data sample comprises 200 cases from the Cardiac Atlas Project (CAP) database [20], of which 100 are healthy subjects and 100 are hearts associated with myocardial infarction. The shapes consist of 3D meshes of the left ventricles at end-diastole and end-systole (two cardiac phases), with point correspondence established previously.

In this work, all the shapes were firstly aligned to remove differences in the coordinates systems between all cases. To achieve this, we aligned all the end-diastole cases and the obtained pose parameters for each case were then applied to the end-systole shape. Differences in scaling were not corrected for as LV size is likely to be an indicator of the disease state. Furthermore, the ED and ES shapes were concatenated into a single shape vector for classification based on Eq. (3).

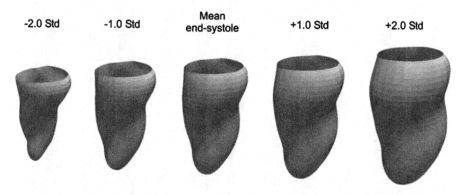

Fig. 1. First mode of variation as obtained from the PLS decomposition for the end-systole shape. It can be seen that the shapes vary from significant motion (−2 Std) that is typical in healthy subjects, all the way up to reduced motion due to infarcted muscle (+2 Std).

Subsequently, we applied the proposed PLS decomposition based on the labels of the datasets (0 for healthy cases, 1 for infarcted hearts). As an illustration, Fig. 1 shows the first mode of variation obtain from the PLS decomposition for the endocardium at end-systole (*i.e.* at maximal muscle contraction), from −2 Std to +2 Std (corresponding to about 98 % of the variability). It can be seen that the shapes vary from significant motion (−2 Std) that is typical in healthy subjects, all the way up to less pronounced cardiac motion due to infarcted muscle (+2 Std). Note that the second and third modes of variation show longitudinal and localized LV motion, respectively, which can also be affected due to myocardial infarction.

3.2   Effect of Latent Variables

To evaluate the strength of the proposed method for the prediction of healthy and infarcted hearts, we must first choose an optimal value for the number of latent variables used in the PLS regression model. In leave-one-out tests with the 200 cases, we varied the number of latent variables using 10 different values (1, 2, 3, 4, 5, 10, 20, 30, 40, and 50) and we then estimated the prediction accuracy for each case. The results plotted in Fig. 2 show that the best predictions are obtained by using between 5 and 15 latent variables (prediction accuracy in the interval 95.0 % to 96.5 %). The maximum prediction accuracy of 96.5 % is obtained for $t = 10$. After 10 latent variables, the prediction accuracy starts to decrease, indicating that the additional shape information does not contribute to the disease state of the subject and even act as noisy information that affect the predictions.

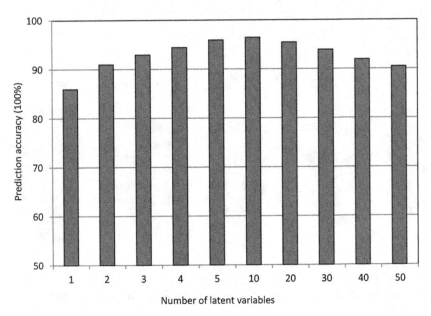

Fig. 2. Effect of number of latent variables on the PLS regression accuracy for the prediction of healthy and infarcted subjects, using leave-one-out tests.

3.3   Effect of Classification Fusion

In this section we evaluate the improvement by fusing different PLS classifiers corresponding to varying numbers of latent variables. Based on the results from previous section, we consider three PLS classifiers obtained by using 5, 10, and 15 latent variables. These three PLS classifiers are then fused using the fusion median method described in Sect. 2.4. The results summarized below in Table 1 show that the classification accuracy improves to 98 % by applying the proposed fusion approach. We

Table 1. Accuracy, specificity, and sensitivity of the different PLS classifiers and their fusion.

PLS classifiers	Accuracy [%]	Specificity [%]	Sensitivity [%]
5 latent variables	95	95	93.5
10 latent variables	96.5	98	96
15 latent variables	95.5	97	94
Fusion	**98**	**99**	**97**

also computed the specificity and sensitivity measures, which also show an improvement in the final results by using the fused PLS classifier of myocardial infarction.

3.4 Effect of Training Size

Finally, we evaluated the effect of training size for the modeling and prediction of healthy/infarcted hearts. We randomly selected an increasing number of datasets (from 20 to 200, in increments of 20) and each time we performed leave-one-out tests. While the results in Fig. 3 indicate that the training size as expected affects the prediction accuracy, it can be also seen that after 100 cases, the improvement is not significant, with prediction accuracy between 94 % for 100 training datasets and 98.0 % for 200 datasets used in the tests. This is because normal hearts differ significantly from infarcted hearts in the morphology (due to remodeling), as well as in the motion (less pronounced contraction). As a result, PLS decomposition with a relatively small training dataset (about 100 cases) is already capable of encoding the differences between healthy and infarcted hearts.

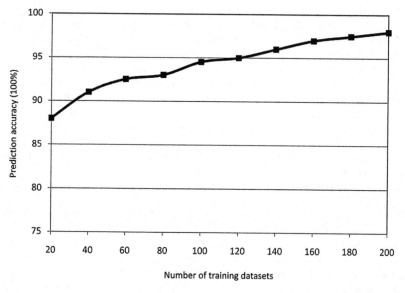

Fig. 3. Effect of the number of datasets used for training the PLS shape models.

4 Conclusions

In this paper we presented an alternative method for the construction of statistical shape models of the left ventricle based on partial least squares (PLS), such that the decomposition is application-specific, *i.e.* it takes into account the diagnostic goal of the study such as to discriminate healthy and infarcted hearts. The results demonstrate promise, with a high prediction accuracy of 98.0 % when using 200 cases in leave-one-out tests.

References

1. Hoogendoorn, C., Duchateau, N., Sánchez-Quintana, D., Whitmarsh, T., Sukno, F., De Craene, M., Lekadir, K., Frangi, A.: A high-resolution atlas and statistical model of the human heart from multislice CT. IEEE Trans. Med. Imaging **32**(1), 28–44 (2013)
2. Hoogendoorn, C., Pashaei, A., Sebastian, R., Sukno, F.M., Cámara, O., Frangi, A.F.: Sensitivity analysis of mesh warping and subsampling strategies for generating large scale electrophysiological simulation data. In: Metaxas, D.N., Axel, L. (eds.) FIMH 2011. LNCS, vol. 6666, pp. 418–426. Springer, Heidelberg (2011)
3. Bosch, J.G., Nijland, F., Mitchell, S.C., Lelieveldt, B.P.F., Kamp, O., Sonka, M., Reiber, J.H.C.: Computer-aided diagnosis via model-based shape analysis: automated classification of wall motion abnormali-ties in echocardiograms. Acad. Radiol. **12**(3), 358–367 (2005)
4. Zhao, F., Zhang, H., Wahle, A., Stolpen, A., Scholz, T., Sonka, M.: Congenital aortic disease: 4D magnetic resonance segmentation and quantitative analysis. Med. Image Anal. **13**(3), 483–493 (2009)
5. Sjoestrand, K., Stegmann, M.B., Larsen, R.: Sparse principal component analysis in medical shape modeling. In: SPIE Medical Imaging: Image Processing (2006)
6. Leung, K., Bosch, J.G.: Localized shape variations for classifying wall motion in echocardiograms. In: Ayache, N., Ourselin, S., Maeder, A. (eds.) MICCAI 2007, Part I. LNCS, vol. 4791, pp. 52–59. Springer, Heidelberg (2007)
7. Lekadir, K., Keenan, N., Pennell, D., Yang, G.Z.: Shape-based myocardial contractility analysis using multivariate outlier detection. In: Ayache, N., Ourselin, S., Maeder, A. (eds.) MICCAI 2007, Part II. LNCS, vol. 4792, pp. 834–841. Springer, Heidelberg (2007)
8. Lekadir, K., Keenan, N., Pennell, D., Yang, G.-Z.: An inter-landmark approach to 4-D shape extraction and interpretation: Application to myocardial motion assessment in MRI. IEEE Trans. Med. Imaging **30**(1), 52–68 (2011)
9. Suinesiaputra, A., Frangi, A.F., Kaandorp, T., Lamb, H.J., Bax, J.J., Reiber, J., Lelieveldt, B.: Automated detection of regional wall motion abnormalities based on a statistical model applied to multislice short-axis cardiac MR images. IEEE Trans. Med. Imaging **28**(4), 595–607 (2009)
10. Wold, S., Geladi, P., Esbensen, K., Öhman, J.: Multi-way principal components-and PLS-analysis. J. Chemometr. **1**(1), 41–56 (1987)
11. Rao, A., Aljabar, P., Rueckert, D.: Hierarchical statistical shape analysis and prediction of sub-cortical brain structures. Med. Image Anal. **12**(1), 55–68 (2008)
12. Lekadir, K., Hoogendoorn, C., Hazrati-Marangalou, J., Taylor, Z., Noble, C., Van Rietbergen, B., Frangi, A.: A predictive model of vertebral trabecular anisotropy from ex vivo micro-CT. IEEE Trans. Med. Imaging **34**, 1747–1759 (2015)

13. Lekadir, K., Pashaei, A., Hoogendoorn, C., Pereanez, M., Alba, X., Frangi, A.F.: Effect of statistically derived fiber models on the estimation of cardiac electrical activation. IEEE Trans. Biomed. Eng. **61**(11), 2740–2748 (2014)
14. Lekadir, K., Hazrati-Marangalou, J., Hoogendoorn, C., Taylor, Z., van Rietbergen, B., Frangi, A.F.: Statistical estimation of femur micro-architecture using optimal shape and density predictors. J. Biomech. **48**(4), 598–603 (2015)
15. Lekadir, K., Hoogendoorn, C., Pereanez, M., Alba, X., Pashaei, A., Frangi, A.F.: Statistical personalization of ventricular fiber orientation using shape predictors. IEEE Trans. Med. Imaging **33**(4), 882–890 (2014)
16. McIntosh, A.R., Lobaugh, N.J.: Partial least squares analysis of neuroimaging data: applications and advances. NeuroImage **23**, S250–S263 (2004)
17. Abdi, H.: Partial least squares regression (PLS-regression), Thousand Oaks, CA, Sage, pp. 792–795 (2003)
18. Pérez-Enciso, M., Tenenhaus, M.: Prediction of clinical outcome with microarray data: a partial least squares discriminant analysis (PLS-DA) approach. Hum. Genet. **112**(5–6), 581–592 (2003)
19. Chevallier, S., Bertrand, D., Kohler, A., Courcoux, P.: Application of PLS-DA in multivariate image analysis. J. Chemometr. **20**(5), 221 (2006)
20. Fonseca, C.G., Backhaus, M., Bluemke, D.A., Britten, R.D., Chung, J.D., Cowan, B.R., Dinov, I.D., Finn, J.P., et al.: The cardiac atlas project–an imaging database for computational modeling and statistical atlases of the heart. Bioinformatics **27**(16), 2288–2295 (2011)

Classification of Myocardial Infarcted Patients by Combining Shape and Motion Features

Wenjia Bai[(✉)], Ozan Oktay, and Daniel Rueckert

Biomedical Image Analysis Group, Department of Computing,
Imperial College London, London, UK
w.bai@imperial.ac.uk

Abstract. Myocardial infarction changes both the shape and motion of the heart. In this work, cardiac shape and motion features are extracted from shape models at ED and ES phases and combined to train a SVM classifier between myocardial infarcted cases and asymptomatic cases. Shape features are characterised by PCA coefficients of a shape model, whereas motion features include wall thickening and wall motion. Evaluated on the STACOM 2015 challenge dataset, the proposed method achieves a high accuracy of 97.5 % for classification, which shows that shape and motion features can be useful biomarkers for myocardial infarction, which provide complementary information to late-gadolinium MR assessment.

1   Introduction

Myocardial infarction results in abrupt increase of loading conditions at both the infarcted and non-infarcted regions of the ventricle. Subsequently, ventricular remodeling occurs which modulates the underlying tissue of the involved regions in order to compensate for the loss of the myocardium and to adapt to the increase of the load [1]. The mechanical function of the ventricular changes accordingly during the process of infarction and post-infarction remodeling.

Clinically, myocardial infarction is assessed using late-gadolinium enhanced MR (LGE-MR) in which the infarcted or fibrotic tissue appears bright due to the reduced clearance and increased volume of distribution of gadolinium, whereas normal tissue appears dark [2]. Since myocardial infarction has a direct impact on anatomical structure and mechanical function, we hypothesise that shape and motion features, derived from non-enhanced cine MR images, can be alternative biomarkers for myocardial infarction. They can provide complementary information to LGE-MR image assessment.

In the past, numerous efforts have been dedicated to cardiac shape analysis [3–5] or cardiac motion analysis [6,7] in the context of cardiomyopathy studies or abnormality detection. Medrano and Perperidis both use PCA for decomposing the cardiac shapes and the PCA coefficients are then used for classification between sub-groups [3,4]. Suinesiaputra instead decomposes the shape at ES using ICA and the ICA coefficients are used for regional wall motion abnormality detection [5]. McLeod estimates motion using a polyaffine LogDemons method,

© Springer International Publishing Switzerland 2016
O. Camara et al. (Eds.): STACOM 2015, LNCS 9534, pp. 140–145, 2016.
DOI: 10.1007/978-3-319-28712-6_15

decomposes the polyaffine parameters spatio-temporally and the decomposition coefficients are used for motion analysis [7]. Duchateau characterises myocardial motion on a spatio-temporally normalised map and assesses the changes of the motion map during bi-ventricular pacing [6].

In this paper, we propose a method for myocardial infarction detection by using combined shape and motion features. On the STACOM 2015 statistical shape modelling challenge dataset, the proposed method has achieved a high accuracy of 97.5 % in detecting patients with myocardial infarction.

2   Methods

2.1   Dataset

In the STACOM 2015 challenge, a training set of 200 cases (100 with myocardial infarction from the DETERMINE cohort, labeled 1; 100 asymptomatic from the MESA cohort, labeled 0) is provided [8]. The provided data include the shape models at ED and ES for each subject. The shape models are generated by fitting a finite-element model to a small amount of user-selected guide points [9]. Bias correction is applied to the shape models afterwards to correct for the protocol-dependent shape bias between the DETERMINE and MESA cohorts [3]. Each shape model contains 1089 vertices on the endocardium and 1089 vertices on the epicardium. The shape models for a testing set of 200 cases (100 infarcted, 100 asymptomatic) are also available, whose labels are unknown to the challenge participants.

2.2   Features

We use two types of features for classification, the myocardial shape features to characterise anatomy and the motion features to characterise mechanical function. We will describe the two type of features subsequently.

Shape. The challenge dataset provides the surface mesh models for all the subjects. To remove position and orientation difference, we compute a mean mesh model and align all the subject meshes to the mean mesh using the rigid registration programme in the IRTK software package[1], which minimises the Euclidean distance between the two point clouds as a least-square problem. For each subject, the rigid transformation is estimated using the mesh at the ED phase. The resulting transformation is then applied to the meshes at both ED and ES phases.

Then principal component analysis (PCA) is performed twice, respectively for all the aligned meshes at the ED phase and then at the ES phase. The PCA coordinates at ED, P_{ED}, and the PCA coordinates at ES, P_{ES}, are used as shape features. We also concatenate the coordinates at two phases to form another shape feature $P = \{P_{ED}, P_{ES}\}$.

---

[1] https://www.doc.ic.ac.uk/~dr/software/.

Motion. The motion information is measured in two aspects, wall thickening and wall displacement. For each vertex on the epicardium, the wall thickness w is measured from this point to the closest point on the endocardium using the FindClosestPoint() function in the VTK library. The closest point can be somewhere on a triangle cell of the mesh, not necessarily to be a vertex. The absolute and relative thickening of the wall from ED to ES are defined by the following equations,

$$T_{abs} = w_{ES} - w_{ED}$$
$$T_{rel} = (w_{ES} - w_{ED})/w_{ED}$$

In addition, wall displacement is computed for each vertex using its coordinate at ED and at ES. The displacement is decomposed into radial, longitudinal and circumferential components using the local cardiac coordinate system [10]. The displacements for both the endocardial and the epicardial vertices are included as features and denoted by $D_{endo,r}$, $D_{endo,l}$, $D_{endo,c}$, $D_{epi,r}$, $D_{epi,l}$ and $D_{epi,c}$. The subscripts r, l and c denote radial, longitudinal and circumferential.

To summarise, 11 feature vectors are extracted, of which 3 encode shape information (P_{ED}, P_{ES} and P) and 8 encode motion information (T_{abs}, T_{rel}, $D_{endo,r}$, $D_{endo,l}$, $D_{endo,c}$, $D_{epi,r}$, $D_{epi,l}$ and $D_{epi,c}$).

2.3 Classifier

A support vector machine (SVM) is trained to classify between the infarcted cases and the asymptomatic cases. The radial basis function (RBF) kernel is chosen, which outperforms the linear kernel in experiments. The default kernel size in the python sklearn library is applied for the RBF kernel, which is the reciprocal of the total number of features[2]. Each of the 11 feature vectors are tested independently as input to the classifier and combinations of the features are also tested. The classification performance is evaluated using 10-fold cross-validation on the training set of 200 cases, repeated for 10 times.

3   Results

3.1   Features

Figure 1 shows the first two PCA coordinates for the 200 training subjects. Clearly, the PCA coordinates contain useful information to tell the difference between the normal and the infarcted. Visually, the two groups seem to have less overlap using the coordinates at ES than using the coordinates at ED.

Figure 2 compares the motion features between a normal subject and an infarcted subject. It shows that for the two exemplar subjects, the normal one has larger displacement magnitude than the infarcted one in basal and mid-ventricular regions.

---

[2] http://scikit-learn.org.

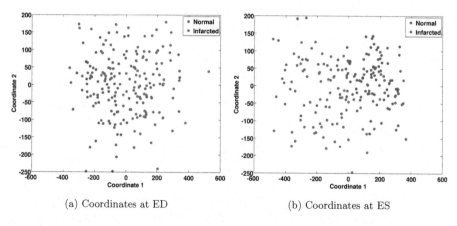

(a) Coordinates at ED   (b) Coordinates at ES

Fig. 1. Plot of the first two PCA coordinates for the 200 training subjects.

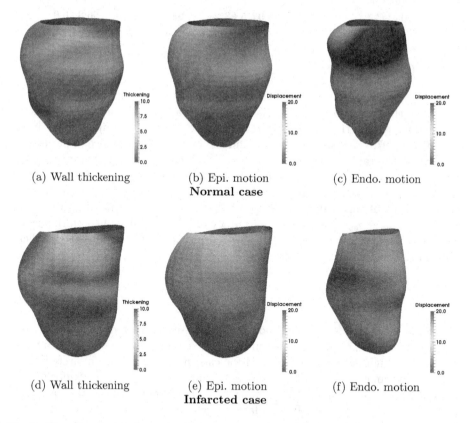

Fig. 2. Visualisation of the motion features for two exemplar subjects (top row: asymptomatic; bottom row: infarcted). The three columns from left to right are respectively absolute wall thickening (unit: mm), epicardial displacement magnitude (unit: mm), endocardial displacement magnitude (unit: mm).

Table 1. Classification performance using each feature independently and using the combination.

Feature		Accuracy (%)	Sensitivity (%)	Specificity (%)
Shape	P_{ED}	92.8±5.2	89.0±9.6	96.6±5.5
	P_{ES}	95.7±4.1	94.0±7.5	97.7±4.6
	P	95.5±4.1	93.0±7.3	**98.0±3.9**
Motion	T_{abs}	92.7±5.5	90.8±9.2	94.3±7.3
	T_{rel}	90.3±6.0	87.7±10.5	92.9±7.9
	$D_{endo,r}$	93.1±5.1	90.9±9.1	95.6±6.2
	$D_{endo,l}$	85.2±7.3	80.7±12.2	90.0±9.7
	$D_{endo,c}$	88.5±6.4	92.3±8.9	85.0±10.6
	$D_{epi,r}$	85.4±8.0	87.0±9.4	84.4±12.3
	$D_{epi,l}$	80.4±8.9	87.5±10.6	73.0±13.7
	$D_{epi,c}$	81.3±8.0	87.6±10.5	75.5±14.1
Combined	$\{P,T_{abs},D_{endo,c},D_{epi,r}\}$	**97.5±3.2**	**98.1±4.2**	96.8±6.0

3.2   Classification Performance

In Table 1, we report the classification performance using each feature independently as the input to the SVM classifier. Accuracy, sensitivity and specificity are evaluated. For the shape features, the first 25 PCA coordinates are used, which keeps 97.0 % of shape variance and shows good performance in parameter tuning. As the table shows, using P_{ES} shows a higher accuracy than using P_{ED}, which is in line with our visual finding from Fig. 1. For the motion features, T_{abs}, $D_{endo,r}$, $D_{endo,c}$ and $D_{epi,r}$ show good performance. We also tested a number of combinations of the shape and motion features and found that the feature set $\{P,T_{abs},D_{endo,c},D_{epi,r}\}$ achieves an accuracy of 97.5 %, which outperforms using each independent feature alone. So we will use this feature set for the classification on the challenge testing set.

4   Conclusions

To conclude, cardiac shape and motion features are extracted from the subject shape models at ED and at ES. When they are combined and used to train a SVM classifier, a high accuracy is achieved for classification between infarcted cases and asymptomatic cases. This could potentially provide valuable information if LGE-MR is not available. A limitation of the current work is that a global classifier is trained for classifying infarction. However, it does not localise where the infarcted region is. A possible extension of the work is to incorporate scar maps into the training set and to train classifiers locally at each region or each vertex so that potentially scar localisation can be achieved using shape and motion features.

References

1. Sutton, M.G.S.J., Sharpe, N.: Left ventricular remodeling after myocardial infarction pathophysiology and therapy. Circulation **101**(25), 2981–2988 (2000)
2. Mandapaka, S., DAgostino, R., Hundley, W.G.: Does late gadolinium enhancement predict cardiac events in patients with ischemic cardiomyopathy? Circulation **113**(23), 2676–2678 (2006)
3. Medrano-Gracia, P., Cowan, B.R., Bluemke, D.A., Finn, J.P., Kadish, A.H., Lee, D.C., Lima, J.A.C., Suinesiaputra, A., Young, A.A.: Atlas-based analysis of cardiac shape and function: correction of regional shape bias due to imaging protocol for population studies. J. Cardiovasc. Magn. Reson. **15**, 80 (2013)
4. Perperidis, D., Mohiaddin, R.H., Rueckert, D.: Construction of a 4D statistical atlas of the cardiac anatomy and its use in classification. In: Duncan, J.S., Gerig, G. (eds.) MICCAI 2005. LNCS, vol. 3750, pp. 402–410. Springer, Heidelberg (2005)
5. Suinesiaputra, A., Frangi, A.F., Kaandorp, T., Lamb, H.J., Bax, J.J., Reiber, J., Lelieveldt, B.P.F.: Automated detection of regional wall motion abnormalities based on a statistical model applied to multislice short-axis cardiac MR images. IEEE Trans. Med. Imaging **28**(4), 595–607 (2009)
6. Duchateau, N., Giraldeau, G., Gabrielli, L., Fernández-Armenta, J., Penela, D., Evertz, R., Mont, L., Brugada, J., Berruezo, A., Sitges, M., et al.: Quantification of local changes in myocardial motion by diffeomorphic registration via currents: Application to paced hypertrophic obstructive cardiomyopathy in 2D echocardiographic sequences. Med. Image Anal. **19**(1), 203–219 (2015)
7. McLeod, K., Sermesant, M., Beerbaum, P., Pennec, X.: Spatio-temporal tensor decomposition of a polyaffine motion model for a better analysis of pathological left ventricular dynamics. In: MICCAI, pp. 501–508. Springer (2013)
8. Fonseca, C.G., Backhaus, M., Bluemke, D.A., Britten, R.D., Chung, J.D., Cowan, B.R., Dinov, I.D., Finn, J.P., Hunter, P.J., Kadish, A.H.: The cardiac atlas project-an imaging database for computational modeling and statistical atlases of the heart. Bioinformatics **27**(16), 2288–2295 (2011)
9. Young, A.A., Cowan, B.R., Thrupp, S.F., Hedley, W.J., DellItalia, L.J.: Left ventricular mass and volume: fast calculation with guide-point modeling on MR images. Radiology **216**(2), 597–602 (2000)
10. Petitjean, C., Rougon, N., Cluzel, P.: Assessment of myocardial function: a review of quantification methods and results using tagged MRI. J. Cardiovasc. Magn. Reson. **7**(2), 501–516 (2005)

Detecting Myocardial Infarction Using Medial Surfaces

LV Statistical Modelling Challenge: Myocardial Infarction

Pierre Ablin and Kaleem Siddiqi[(✉)]

School of Computer Science and Centre for Intelligent Machines,
McGill University, Montreal, Canada
Siddiqi@cim.mcgill.ca

Abstract. The shape of the heart is known to undergo significant alteration as a result of myocardial infarction. We hypothesize that the thickness of the heart wall is an important variable in discriminating normal hearts from those with such defects. In the context of the present statistical modeling challenge, with meshes provided to describe the epicardium and endocardium at end diastole (ED) and end systole (ES), we model local heart wall thickness using a medial surface representation of fixed single sheet topology. Such a surface lies between the heart walls and the radius of the maximal inscribed disk at each point on it reveals heart wall thickness. We align the ED and ES medial surfaces to one another using the coherent point drift algorithm, and then align each registered pair to that of a reference heart, so that locations within each medial surface are in spatial correspondence with one another. We then treat the radius values at these corresponding medial surface point locations as inputs to a support vector machine. Our experiments yield a 96 % correct detection rate on the 200 cases of labeled test data, demonstrating the promise of this approach.

1 Introduction

The STACOM 2015 challenge involves distinguishing hearts which have suffered from myocardial infarction from those that are normal, given only 3D shape information. The input data from Fonseca et al. [1] are Cartesian point sets describing the epicardium and the endocardium at ED and ES, along with triangulation information for each surface, allowing each to be represented as a mesh. No information is provided about myofiber arrangement, cell density, myocardial mass, or the age of the infarct when present.

The mechanisms that are involved in the remodelling of the heart as a consequence of an infarction are complex. For example, Weisman et al. suggest that the heart wall gets thinner around the zone where the infarct has occurred, and that the left ventricle (LV) loses its circular shape [2]. Litwin et al. discuss the process of LV remodelling after an infarction and point out that infarcted hearts tend to be thinner [3]. They also discuss how other parameters such as fractional shortening and filling velocity are affected. Sutton et al. explain how the infarct

© Springer International Publishing Switzerland 2016
O. Camara et al. (Eds.): STACOM 2015, LNCS 9534, pp. 146–153, 2016.
DOI: 10.1007/978-3-319-28712-6_16

zone propagates over time, showing that it may take months before the remodeling ends and a balance is found [4]. Taken together, past research suggests that classifying myocardial infarction from 3D shape alone is a tall order. The test cases that are infarcted in the STACOM challenge are likely not all at the same stage of remodeling. In the early stages that follow an infarction, the infarcted zone is well defined as a small tissue necrosis zone, but the heart eventually reshapes itself in a way that makes this zone more difficult to localize.

Despite these difficulties, there is consensus in the literature that structural changes to the myocardium following an infarct are highly correlated with heart wall thickness. Motivated by this observation, we propose to measure local heart wall thickness using a medial surface representation and to use it to perform both within subject and between subject registration of hearts. We describe our processing pipeline to compute medial surfaces in Sect. 2 and then explain how we treat the associated radius function as data for use by a machine learning method for classification in Sect. 3. In Sect. 4 we describe the machine learning algorithms that we have used, and present our results on the test data. We conclude with a discussion of the strengths and weaknesses of our method in Sect. 5.

2   Computing the Medial Surfaces

The medial surface or the 3D skeleton is comprised of the locus of centres of maximal inscribed disks within a volumetric object, along with the associated radius values. First introduced by Blum in [5] medial representations have been widely used in computer vision, robotics, medical imaging and other domains because they provide a compact representation of an object while facilitating shape analysis. In the continuum this representation is lossless because an object can be reconstructed as the union of balls of appropriate radii centered on the medial surface. The mathematics of this representation is rich and is now well understood, and algorithms for computing it along with many applications are mature [6]. As an illustration, Fig. 1 shows a medial surface comprised of a single sheet describing the wall of a left ventricle. Here the points on the medial surface are colored according to local thickness, i.e., radius of the maximal inscribed disk.

The medial surface can have complex branching sheet topology, which is related to the number and location of curvature maxima (ridges) on the object's surface. In the present application we wish to explicitly relate the epicardium and endocardium at both ED and ES to one another via a single sheet, motivated by the observation that the heart wall is smooth. Inspired by the average outward flux approach of Chap. 4 in [6], we opt for a more direct approach for the particular case of the left ventricle.

Our first step is to obtain a representation of the LV wall using a voxelization method. We scale every heart to have a constant diameter during ED, while storing the scaling coefficients as they might prove useful for classification. We also rotate each heart in order to have its major axis aligned with the x-axis. We then voxelize the heart wall surfaces, with a resolution that guarantees that

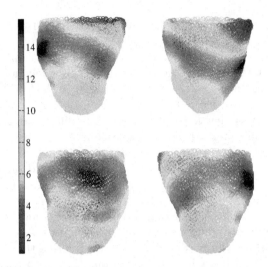

Fig. 1. A medial surface computed for the wall of a left ventricle, viewed from four different angles. The colors indicate the local thickness of the wall in voxel units (Color figure online).

every point on the epicardial and endocardial mesh surfaces lies in one and only one voxel. Once this is done, we proceed to voxelize the outer wall and the inner wall surfaces using the provided triangulation files, while leaving no holes. We then use a recursive seed filling algorithm on a capped version of each heart. The capping is accomplished via a plane having equation $x = K$, where K is chosen to prevent leaking while retaining as many points as possible. Subtracting the set of voxels within the endocardial volume from those within the epicardial volume then leaves the set of voxels lying within the LV myocardial wall.

Following this, [6] suggests to compute the Euclidean distance function between the wall surface and each point within the interior of the object. The idea is then to compute the average outward flux through a small sphere around each point of the distance function gradient. In theory, this quantity is non zero only on the medial surface that we are seeking, but we are dealing with numerical approximations that make this approach require some parameter tuning. In the present article we opt for a more direct method since we wish to obtain a single medial surface with non-branching topology. Given that we have direct access to both heart walls, we compute the distance functions to these two surfaces separately, and treat the medial points as those where these two functions have the same value.

Figure 2 provides a summary of our processing pipeline. In practice we compute for each voxel v within the LV wall the absolute value of the difference between its distances to the two walls: $f(v) = |d_{outer}(v) - d_{inner}(v)|$, and find its zeros. Figure 2(b) shows a plot of f on an axial slice of a left ventricle. Overall, this process leads to smooth, thin medial surfaces.

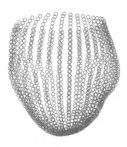

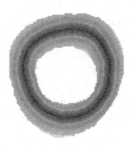

(a) The initial point set data. Here the epicardial wall of one LV during ED is displayed.

(b) A plot of the function f on an axial slice of the filled myocardial wall. The deep blue zone is where f is almost zero, indicating the locus of points on the medial surface.

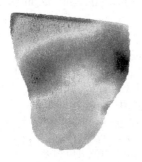

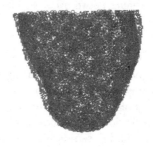

(c) The medial surface. Color denotes thickness according to the color bar in Fig. 1.

(d) Two distinct medial surfaces are aligned using the coherent point drift algorithm.

Fig. 2. Our processing pipeline. We first obtain a voxelized heart wall and compute the function f within it, from which we extract the medial surface. Each ED medial surface is then registered to the ES medial surface, following which all ED medial surfaces are registered to a single reference ED medial surface.

3   Registering the Medial Surfaces

For each heart, we now have two medial surfaces, one corresponding to ED and one to ES, where the thickness of the heart wall is encoded in the medial surface radius value at each location on it. In order to observe the change of thickness during the heartbeat, we must find a correspondence map between the ED and ES surfaces. We have previously centered and scaled each heart, but we cannot assume that the input hearts are perfectly aligned. To perform registration, we opt for the coherent point drift algorithm presented in [7] because it is fast, accurate, noise resistant and gives smooth correspondences. It also does not require an explicit triangulation of either surface. To speed up the process we sub-sample each medial surface, randomly picking 5000 points on it. Registration gives us a function $p : \{1 ; 5000\} \rightarrow \{1 ; 5000\}$, such that the ith point of the ED medial surface corresponds to the $p(i)^{th}$ point of the ES medial surface. This allows us to visualize the wall thickening, as displayed in Fig. 3.

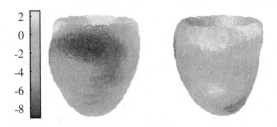

Fig. 3. Wall thickening between ED and ES, shown from two different viewing directions on a medial surface.

Our initial hope was that this representation would give us a simple way to discriminate between hearts with infarctions and normal ones. For instance, infarcted zones might be reflected by an unusual local wall thickening. In practice it turns out that both the normal and the infarcted hearts have zones of thickness change, with no obvious way to distinguish one from the other. Infarcted hearts tend to have a smaller radius change on average, and most show zones that get thicker during diastole, but some normal hearts also have this property. We decided to describe every heart via an ordered list of medial surface radius values during both ES and ED and to use a higher level machine learning process for classification via a labeled test set. In order to be able to compare wall thickness between hearts it was necessary to first match corresponding locations between them, i.e., the first radius that we pick to describe the first heart must geometrically correspond to the first radius of every other heart. To do so, we pick one ED medial surface as a reference, and compute the correspondence map of each heart's medial surfaces during ED and ES with this reference. The following schematic shows how each heart's medial surface radius values are stored:

$$\text{Heart 1} \rightarrow \quad r^1_{ED,1} \quad r^1_{ES,1} \quad r^1_{ED,2} \quad \cdots \quad r^1_{ED,5000} \quad r^1_{ES,5000}$$

$$\text{Heart n} \rightarrow \quad r^n_{ED,1} \quad r^n_{ES,1} \quad r^n_{ED,2} \quad \cdots \quad r^n_{ED,5000} \quad r^n_{ES,5000}$$

Each column of the above matrix contains the radius values of medial surface points which correspond to one another in terms of their spatial location. In other words $r_{ED,1}^1$, $r_{ED,1}^2$, ... , $r_{ED,1}^n$ are the radii of distinct ED medial surfaces at a location which is in correspondence between them. The columns are not ordered in any particular way and we would obtain the same classification results if we were to shuffle them.

4 Statistical Analysis

We provide the list of medial surface radius values in spatial correspondence with one another as inputs to machine learning algorithms. This data contains meaningful information about heart wall thickness since the medial surfaces have been co-registered. The best results we have been able to obtain so far on the test data set are via the application of a simple support vector machine (SVM) algorithm, as suggested by [8]. We first use principal component analysis to reduce the number of features from 10000 (5000 radius values for ED and 5000 for ES) to 100. We then use a radial basis kernel function SVM to classify our hearts. With the right choice of parameters, we obtain promising results. In particular, using k-fold cross validation, with a k of 40 (i.e. 20 % of our dataset) we obtain an accuracy of 96 % correct classification on average. Some hearts appear to cause more trouble than others. For example, for the 200 labelled test cases we have, cross validation *always* classifies 171 hearts correctly. 14 other hearts are accurately classified over 90 % of the time while 9 other hearts have a classification error rate under 40 %. The 6 remaining hearts are almost always misclassified. A histogram of misclassification rates is shown in Fig. 4.

We also experimented with a random forest algorithm, as described in [9], to compare its performance against the SVM. It achieves promising accuracy results (88 %) but does not perform quite as well as the SVM algorithm. Interestingly enough, the random forest approach yields the same classification errors as the SVM when it comes to the 6 problematic cases. This suggests a limitation of

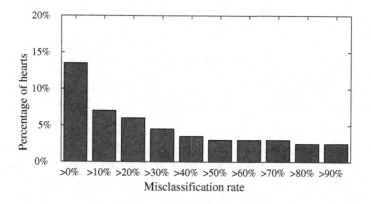

Fig. 4. Histogram of the misclassification rate over multiple cross validation experiments. Most of the hearts are almost always correctly classified, but a small proportion is not.

diagnostic information in wall thickness as measured by medial surface radius values, rather than an inherent limitation of the classification method itself.

5   Discussion

Our results demonstrate that relating the epicardium to the endocardium explicitly via a medial surface has potential for detecting myocardial infarction. This representation provides direct access to both shape and thickness information. Qualitatively the merits of this approach can be seen simply by observing the average radii of the medial surfaces (which excludes all the topological and geometrical information that they also contain). This is illustrated in Fig. 5 via a scatter plot in which each heart is represented by a 2D point (x, y), where x is the mean medial radius of a heart during ED and y is its mean medial radius during ES. The points in blue correspond to the infarcted hearts in the test data, while the points in red correspond to the normal hearts. Although some points are interleaved, the red and blue clusters are quite well separated.

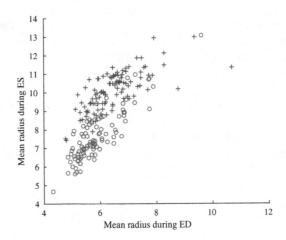

Fig. 5. Each heart is represented by a 2D point whose coordinates are the mean radii of the medial surface during ED and ES. Although the separation is not perfect, it is qualitatively quite good. The red circles correspond to normal hearts and the blue crosses to ones with infarcts. The radii are in voxel units (Color figure online).

As discussed earlier, an infarction leads to complex changes in the thickness of the heart wall. Our first hope was that an infarcted heart would show some dead zones that would have an approximately constant thickness over time. To test this hypothesis, we registered the ED and ES medial surfaces together, and then plotted the radius change between these two phases for each point on the medial surface. In practice it turns out that both normal and infarcted hearts contain such zones, with no obvious way to distinguish one from the other. While wall thickening is an important diagnostic parameter, other geometric features could also be taken account, such as the local shape and curvature of the heart wall. A limitation of our approach is that we have not taken the direction of wall thickening into account, i.e., be it due to dilation of the epicardium or due to contraction of the endocardium.

We have also experimented with using medial surface point locations as additional features to the machine learning classification algorithms and as well with averaging radius values over a small local neighborhood on the medial surface. Neither of these strategies have boosted classification performance, likely because the medial surface points are co-registered and the medial surface radius values vary smoothly. Despite its present limitations, using machine learning approaches on the radius values of co-registered ED and ES medial surfaces yields promising classification results on the test data.

References

1. Fonseca, C.G., Backhaus, M., Bluemke, D.A., Britten, R.D., Chung, J.D., Cowan, B.R., Dinov, I.D., Finn, J.P., Hunter, P.J., Kadish, A.H., et al.: The cardiac atlas projectan imaging database for computational modeling and statistical atlases of the heart. Bioinformatics **27**, 2288–2295 (2011)
2. Weisman, H.F., Bush, D.E., Mannisi, J.A., Weisfeldt, M.L., Healy, B.: Cellular mechanisms of myocardial infarct expansion. Circulation **78**, 186–201 (1988)
3. Litwin, S.E., Katz, S.E., Morgan, J.P., Douglas, P.S.: Serial echocardiographic assessment of left ventricular geometry and function after large myocardial infarction in the rat. Circulation **89**, 345–354 (1994)
4. Sutton, M.G.S.J., Sharpe, N.: Left ventricular remodeling after myocardial infarction pathophysiology and therapy. Circulation **101**, 2981–2988 (2000)
5. Blum, H.: Biological shape and visual science (part i). J. Theor. Biol. **38**, 205–287 (1973)
6. Siddiqi, K., Pizer, S.: Medial Representations: Mathematics, Algorithms and Applications. Springer Science & Business Media, Netherlands (2008)
7. Myronenko, A., Song, X.: Point set registration: coherent point drift. IEEE Trans. Pattern Anal. Mach. Intell. **32**, 2262–2275 (2010)
8. Hsu, C.W., Chang, C.C., Lin, C.J., et al.: A practical guide to support vector classification (2003)
9. Breiman, L.: Random forests. Mach. Learn. **45**, 5–32 (2001)

Left Ventricle Classification Using Active Shape Model and Support Vector Machine

Nripesh Parajuli[1]([✉]), Allen Lu[2], and James S. Duncan[1,2,3]

[1] Department of Electrical Engineering, Yale University, New Haven, CT, USA
nripesh.parajuli@yale.edu
[2] Department of Biomedical Engineering, Yale University, New Haven, CT, USA
[3] Department of Diagnostic Radiology, Yale University, New Haven, CT, USA

Abstract. We present the methods and results of building an Active Shape Model (ASM) of the left ventricle (LV) and using a Support Vector Machine (SVM) learning model to classify normal and infarcted LVs provided in the STACOM 2015 Statistical Shape Analysis Challenge dataset. First, all LVs are rigidly registered to a reference LV. In this way, the entire dataset is aligned to the same reference frame. Then, the shape model is obtained by Principal Component Analysis (PCA) decomposition of the aligned LVs. This allows us to capture the principal modes of variation in the LV shapes and reduce the dimensionality of our data.

Next, we train an SVM learning model on our data. To test the performance of the model before using it on the unlabeled test set, we test our method by partitioning the dataset with labels into a training set and a test set of equal sizes. We train the model only using the training set and predict the labels of the test set we created (whose labels were known but not used during training). We repeated this for 100 different random partitions and achieved 94 % prediction accuracy with 94 % sensitivity and 93 % specificity on the test set.

Keywords: Shape modeling · Active shape model · Support vector machine · Classification

1 Introduction

The task of building a shape based statistical model of the LV is challenging. Representation of the LV shape is not uniform across literature. The nature of intensity images of the heart varies significantly across imaging devices, conditions and modalities. If acquired images are not physiologically consistent, for instance if they do not capture the same region from the base to apex of the heart, it is difficult to align them correctly to build a statistical model.

The STACOM 2015 challenge dataset consisted of 200 DETERMINE (disease cases, [1]) and 200 MESA (normal cases, [2]) LV point clouds (along with their finite element models) contributed to the Cardiac Atlas Project (CAP) [3]. Of these, half of them were labeled and the other half were not.

O. Camara et al. (Eds.): STACOM 2015, LNCS 9534, pp. 154–161, 2016.
DOI: 10.1007/978-3-319-28712-6_17

Just as the rest of the CAP aims to build structural and functional atlases of the heart, and in the process, help develop and benchmark diverse cardiac modeling and statistical techniques, this challenge also provided a unique opportunity to attempt to model the cardiac shape characteristics and build an algorithm to detect myocardial infarction. Given that cardiovascular diseases are the largest contributing factors to mortality in the developed world, a robust and well validated detection technique of myocardial infarction could be of great value scientifically and clinically.

In this work we build a shape model using ASM, first proposed by Cootes et al. in [4]. In this particular formulation, the shape space is first decomposed into a lower dimension using PCA. The data is projected onto the eigenspace derived from the PCA of the training set. The test data's projection will then adhere to the variation found in the training set. This serves as a form of shape prior.

Then, the PCA coefficients are used as features for the SVM classification model. The number of features, the width of the RBF kernel and the data adherence term C of the SVM are chosen using 10-fold cross validation.

2   Methods

2.1   Alignment of Shape Data

The Procrustes method is used to align all LVs to a reference LV. First, a random end diastolic (ED) LV is chosen as reference. Then all other ED LVs are aligned to the reference ED LV. This is done by solving for a transformation consisting of rotation, translation and scaling that minimizes the mean square distance between the reference and the shape to be aligned. Then the mean ED LV shape is calculated by taking the mean of all aligned corresponding shape points. All shapes are then again registered with the mean shape.

This is repeated 25 times, by randomly choosing 25 different ED LVs as the starting reference. The mean shape formed by using a reference that led to the lowest mean square error overall was retained as the mean shape (Fig. 1).

Finally, all ED LVs are registered to the chosen mean LV. Assuming that ED and end systolic (ES) frames for same patients are already aligned, the

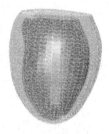

Fig. 1. Mean End Diastole (ED) Left Ventricle (LV)

transformation that maps any given ED frame to the mean ED LV is also applied to the ES. This is done to ensure that they are both aligned to the mean LV while their relative differences, which must be retained, are preserved under a linear transformation.

2.2   Shape Model

We have n data points in our training set, where each data point $x \in \mathbb{R}^{1 \times p}$ ($p = 13068$ in our model). Since we concatenate all ED and ES LV points as one vector, we get 6534 features from both ED and ES (including endocardial and epicardial, both of which have 1089 points with x, y and z components each).

PCA is carried out on this feature set. A matrix $W = (w_1, w_2, w_3, \ldots w_k)^\intercal$ of principal component coefficients is obtained, where each $w_i \in \mathbb{R}^{p \times 1}$ and k is the chosen number of principal components. The matrix W maps any given data point x to its principal component score $t \in \mathbb{R}^{1 \times k}$ using:

$$x' = x - \bar{x}$$
$$t = x'W \tag{1}$$

Where $\bar{x}$ is the mean of the training feature set. Later when a feature set x from the test set is to processed, it is projected in the same eigenspace by following the same method (Fig. 2).

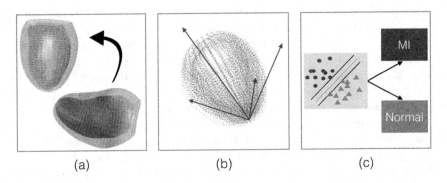

(a)   (b)   (c)

Fig. 2. Method steps: (a) Alignment of a shape (green) to mean shape (red) (b) PCA of aligned shapes (c) SVM classification into normal vs myocardial infarction (MI) (Color figure online)

We qualitatively validate whether or not the eigenspace decomposition captures the natural variation existing in the dataset. This is done by using the method of Cootes et al. where new shapes are generated by adding the principal components multiplied by different amounts to the mean shape and checking the responses [4]. For instance, to see the variations captured by the first principal component, we add the following quantity to the mean shape:

$$x_{new} = \bar{x} + \lambda_1 w_1 \tag{2}$$

-2α ←————————————————————————→ 2α

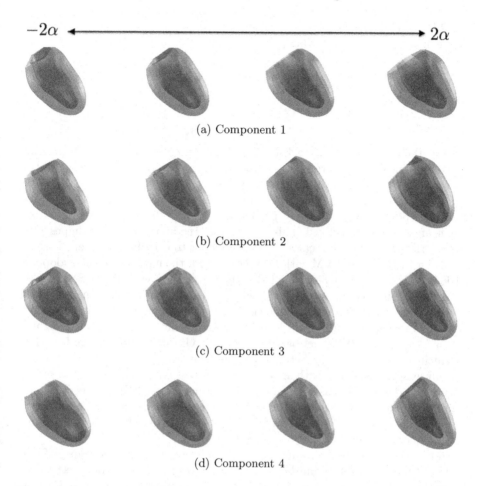

(a) Component 1

(b) Component 2

(c) Component 3

(d) Component 4

Fig. 3. Variation from the mean LV observed by adding first 4 principal components to it.

λ_i is proportional to the variance α_i of the ith principal component. We choose $\lambda_i = (-2\alpha_i, \alpha_i, \alpha_i, 2\alpha_i)$. In Fig. 3, we show how just the first four components have managed to capture significant variation in the shape property of the LV at ES (around 50 % variance). We typically use 15–20 components for our final model.

2.3 SVM Classification

After dimensionality reduction using PCA, we use the soft-margin formulation of the SVM algorithm proposed by Cortes and Vapnik [5] with Radial Basis Function (RBF) kernels. Now assuming $\mathbf{x}$ as the data point already projected into the PCA eigenspace, we have the following classification problem:

$$\mathcal{D} = \{(\mathbf{x}_i, y_i) \mid \mathbf{x}_i \in \mathbb{R}^p, \, y_i \in \{-1, 1\}\}_{i=1}^{n} \tag{3}$$

$\mathcal{D}$ is our training set and $y_i = -1$ for normal cases and $y_i = 1$ for infarction. We then carry out the following optimization:

$$\arg \min_{\mathbf{w},\xi,b} \left\{ \frac{1}{2}\|\mathbf{w}\|^2 + C_i \sum_{i=1}^{n} \xi_i \right\}$$

$$\text{subject to } (\forall i \in \{1,n\}) :$$

$$y_i(\mathbf{w} \cdot \mathbf{K}(\mathbf{x_i}, \mathbf{x_i}') - b) \geq 1 - \xi_i, \quad \xi_i \geq 0$$

(4)

$\mathbf{w}$ is the weight of the RBF kernels and C_i is the data adherence term. This is the well known soft-margin kernel based SVM optimization equation and the convex dual form of this problem is solved [5].

A slight modification is made here by using a variable weight $C_i = c * \Delta_i$ for each data points. Δ_i is inversely proportional to the distance of a shape from the mean shape and c is fixed. This is done with the hypothesis that shapes with large variations from the mean shape are difficult to classify accurately.

As for the choice of SVM with RBF kernels, for the method we have adopted, RBF kernel based SVM performed slightly better than with linear SVM (.93). However, it is interesting to note that, when we carried out the alignment process by only rigidly registering the endocardiums (and applying the same transformation to the epicardiums), we found that the linear SVM performed slightly better (.94) than RBF kernel based SVM (.93). Of further note is the fact that specificity (.95) was slightly better than sensitivity (.93).

Our hypothesis is that with an alignment process based only on endocardium (where the deformation is higher), the RBF kernel based SVM overfitted the training data and the linear SVM achieved the appropriate balance. The opposite is potentially true in the case of alignment with entire LV where the epicardium with smaller deformation is also included.

Since the differences were minimal, it is difficult to justify the choice of one SVM method over another but because RBF kernels provided slightly better sensitivity, we chose it over linear SVM since in a clinical setting higher sensitivity might be more desirable.

During our experimentation with different parameters, we found that the choice of C, the kernel scale parameter ψ (the width of the radial basis function) and the number of features used (the number of principal components used from PCA) were critical. We carried out 10-fold cross validation on a number of combinations of these parameters to choose the best set. Figure 4 shows a representative case of how the parameters affect the training error rate during cross validation. Smaller k values seem more stable but also have more error in average. For C and ψ, the errors are low and consistent towards the middle of their respective ranges as expected.

3   Results

3.1   Primary Analysis

We first present results for the straightforward train-test cycle. The training data with labels (normal $= 0$, infarction $= 1$) is partitioned into a training set and

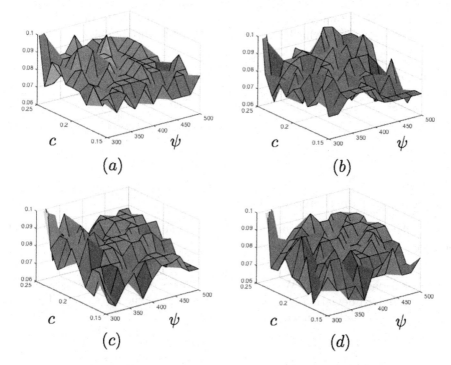

Fig. 4. Error distribution for varying parameters C, ψ and k(number of PCA components) with (a) $k = 12$, (b) $k = 15$, (c) $k = 18$ and (d) $k = 21$.

a test set of equal sizes (100 and 100). The prediction accuracy for the training and the test sets, along with sensitivity (true positives) and specificity (true negatives) are shown in Table 1.

Table 1. Prediction accuracy.

	Accuracy	Sensitivity	Specificity
Training	.96 ± .017	.97 ± .024	.96 ± .026
Test	.94 ± .026	.94 ± .051	.93 ± .043

3.2 Effects of Varying Training Data Size

We first explore how prediction accuracies are affected when training data size is altered. Table 2 summarizes the analysis. It is interesting to note that there is very little difference in accuracy when training size goes from 60 % to 80 %. This either means roughly half of the data was enough to capture the total variation present in the data (and adding more didn't provide any extra information) or there is room for improvement in the shape or the learning model.

Table 2. Accuracy for different training data size (as % of total data size).

Training size, % =	20	40	60	80
	$.64 \pm .10$	$.92 \pm .032$	$.94 \pm .019$	$.94 \pm 0.015$

3.3 Effects of Perturbation on Data

We simulate different scenarios where the LV shape data can be corrupt and how that affects the performance of our model.

Noise on Position Data. We first show the effects of adding gaussian noise of varying standard deviation (σ) to the position data of the LV shapes. The test accuracies are presented in Table 3.

Table 3. Accuracy after adding noise, mislabeling and misalignment.

Noise, σ =	1	2	4	8
	$.92 \pm .024$	$.88 \pm .036$	$.71 \pm .084$	$.52 \pm 0.17$
Mislabeing, % =	5	10	20	40
	$.93 \pm .028$	$.92 \pm .037$	$.81 \pm .066$	$.58 \pm 0.18$
Misalignment, % =	5	10	20	40
	$.91 \pm .026$	$.82 \pm .040$	$.60 \pm .054$	$.47 \pm .019$

We can see how performance remains stable until $\sigma = 2$. At higher levels of noise, it is difficult to form accurate shape models and performance declines.

Mislabeling. Next, we observe how performance is affected if training data is wrongly labeled. We randomly mislabel different percentages of training data points and record the prediction accuracy of the test set as shown in Table 3.

When the mislabeling percentage is high, the performance declines steeply. We compared this result with that of an unsupervised learning method, which is agnostic to training labels. For higher than 10 % mislabeling, k-means clustering (with $k = 2$) performed better (with >90 % accuracy).

Misalignment. Finally, we misalign certain percentage of each data. Since we operated on the point cloud as is, assuming that the data is approximately physiologically aligned, we wanted to explore what happens when some of that consistency is perturbed. The misalignment is simply done by randomly reordering certain data points. Results are presented in Table 3.

Here again, small amount of misalignment does not seem to dramatically reduce performance. However, at higher misalignment percentages, the performance is highly affected. Although not shown here, the training accuracies were much higher than testing accuracies, indicating some possibility of overfitting.

4   Conclusion

We have observed that the combination of ASM based shape modeling and SVM classification has allowed us to build a simple yet effective model to identify LV shapes with and without myocardial infarction. We consistently achieved good results by testing our method by splitting the provided training data into two halves.

We tested our model by changing the training data size and simulating noise, mislabeling and misalignment in the data. For small quantities of noise and small percentages of mislabeling and misalignment, our results were not significantly affected. Also, we achieved the same level of accuracy for training data size of 80 % and 60 %.

We also compared our results with that of an unsupervised learning method (k-means). For most cases, our supervised learning method performed better. Only during the presence of mislabeling, the unsupervised method performed better, which is to be expected since unsupervised learning does not take data labels into account.

Overall, we believe that the ASM based shape modeling along with SVM classification is robust with very good performance.

References

1. Kadish, A.H., Bello, D., Finn, J., Bonow, R.O., Schaechter, A., Subacius, H., Albert, C., Daubert, J.P., Fonseca, C.G., Goldberger, J.J.: Rationale and design for the defibrillators to reduce risk by magnetic resonance imaging evaluation (determine) trial. J. Cardiovasc. Electrophysiol. **20**, 982–987 (2009)
2. Bild, D.E., Bluemke, D.A., Burke, G.L., Detrano, R., Roux, A.V.D., Folsom, A.R., Greenland, P., Jacobs Jr., D.R., Kronmal, R., Liu, K., et al.: Multi-ethnic study of atherosclerosis: objectives and design. Am. J. Epidemiol. **156**, 871–881 (2002)
3. Fonseca, C.G., Backhaus, M., Bluemke, D.A., Britten, R.D., Do Chung, J., Cowan, B.R., Dinov, I.D., Finn, J.P., Hunter, P.J., Kadish, A.H., et al.: The cardiac atlas projectan imaging database for computational modeling and statistical atlases of the heart. Bioinformatics **27**, 2288–2295 (2011)
4. Cootes, T.F., Taylor, C.J., Cooper, D.H., Graham, J.: Active shape models-their training and application. Comput. Vis. Image Underst. **61**, 38–59 (1995)
5. Cortes, C., Vapnik, V.: Support-vector networks. Mach. Learn. **20**, 273–297 (1995)

Supervised Learning of Functional Maps for Infarct Classification

Anirban Mukhopadhyay[1], Ilkay Oksuz[2(✉)], and Sotirios A. Tsaftaris[2,3]

[1] Zuse Institute Berlin, Berlin, Germany
[2] IMT Institute for Advanced Studies Lucca, Lucca, Italy
ilkay.oksuz@imtlucca.it
[3] Department of Electrical Engineering and Computer Science,
Northwestern University, Evanston, USA

Abstract. Our submission to the STACOM Challenge at MICCAI 2015 is based on the supervised learning of functional map representation between End Systole (ES) and End Diastole (ED) phases of Left Ventricle (LV), for classifying infarcted LV from the healthy ones. The Laplace-Beltrami eigen-spectrum of the LV surfaces at ES and ED, represented by their triangular meshes, are used to compute the functional maps. Multi-scale distortions induced by the mapping, are further calculated by singular value decomposition of the functional map. During training, the information of whether an LV surface is healthy or diseased is known, and this information is used to train an SVM classifier for the singular values at multiple scales corresponding to the distorted areas augmented with surface area difference of epicardium and endocardium meshes. At testing similar augmented features are calculated and fed to the SVM model for classification. Promising results are obtained on both cross validation of training data as well as on testing data, which encourages us in believing that this algorithm will perform favourably in comparison to state of the art methods.

Keywords: Infarct · Cardiac remodeling · Laplace-Beltrami · SVM · SVD

1 Introduction

Cardiac remodeling is a clinical term to refer the geometric changes occur on the Left Ventricle (LV) due to myocardial infarction. This phenomenon is considered as an important predictor for survival [14] in clinical practice. However current clinical practices are limited to simple quantities like mass, volume, dimension ratio etc. for important predictions. As a result, important geometric quantities are completely ignored in clinical practice, and only few recent studies on small population have been proposed to quantitatively measure the geometrical structural modification of LV during cardiac remodeling in Multirow Detector Computer Tomography (MDCT) images [8–10].

© Springer International Publishing Switzerland 2016
O. Camara et al. (Eds.): STACOM 2015, LNCS 9534, pp. 162–170, 2016.
DOI: 10.1007/978-3-319-28712-6_18

However, large population-based studies have been recently performed using cardiovascular magnetic resonance (CMR) imaging [2]. CMR, as a non-invasive radiation-free modality, provides rich and detailed quantitative data of the cardiac function and structure. The main goal of the STACOM 2015 challenge is to employ shape analysis and pattern recognition techniques to quantitatively measure geometric changes during cardiac remodeling. In this paper, rather than approaching the problem in a pure feature-driven binary classification technique, we aimed quantifying and visualizing the shape deformation between End Systolic (ES) and End Diastolic (ED) states for healthy and diseased LVs.

Cardiac remodeling results in contraction of myocardium and volume. When represented as a 2D manifold embedded in 3D space, these quantities can be approximated by the surface area of the 2D manifold discretized as a triangular mesh. As a result, a measure of surface area distortion can effectively quantify cardiac remodeling. Moreover, we have also observed that the area distortion of LV is a multi-scale phenomenon and tried to model it in a similar multi-scale fashion (from global to local) to emphasize actual physiological changes. In terms of machine learning, these steps can be considered as a feature selection procedure which ensures the selection of most distinguishing features. In particular, we have incorporated the recently developed functional map framework [11,12] to analyze and visualize ES-ED shape variation between healthy and diseased LVs.

We hypothesize that by learning the features of those regions, where the ES-ED deformation has introduced maximum distortion, we can successfully quantify the geometric changes during cardiac remodeling. The main contributions of this paper are twofold. First, we introduce Functional Map based shape variation exploration in cardiac image analysis context. Second, we present supervised learning of localized feature variations for quantifying cardiac remodeling. The remainder of the paper is organized as follows: Sect. 2 discusses related work, Sect. 3 presents the proposed method, whereas the implementation details are described in Sect. 4. Results are described in Sect. 5 and finally, Sect. 6 offers discussions and conclusion.

2   Related Work

Finite-element analysis has been the de-facto standard for modeling LV shape and function, providing measures accurate enough to be incorporated into clinical practice [7]. Principal component analysis (PCA) is extensively used for analyzing the modes of shape patterns found in populations [1]. However, the unsupervised nature of PCA is sometimes limited towards finding clinically interpretable features.

The most advanced technique for quantifying geometric changes during cardiac remodeling is proposed by Mukhopadhyay et al. in this series of work [8–10]. Here, the authors have proposed 3D Bag-of-words approach with extrinsic and intrinsic isometry invariant geometric features for quantifying local cardiac remodeling. However, this work does not address the multi-scale properties of distortion introduced by cardiac remodeling.

3   Method

In the proposed approach, we have relied on derived quantities of functional maps, in order to learn the distortions introduced during cardiac remodeling. Before describing the proposed approach in detail, we provided an overview of the functional map framework proposed by Ovsjanikov et al. [11] in Sect. 3.1 and the distortion analysis mechanism [12] in Sect. 3.2.

3.1   Functional Maps

A functional map is a novel approach for inference and manipulation of maps between shapes that tries to resolve the issues of correspondences in a fundamentally different manner. Rather than plotting the corresponding points on the shapes, the mappings between functions defined on the shapes are considered. This notion of correspondence generalizes the standard point-to-point map since every point-wise correspondence induces a mapping between function spaces, while the opposite, in general, is not true.

The proposed functional map framework described above provides an elegant way, using a functional representation, to avoid direct representation of correspondences as mappings between shapes. Ovsjanikov et al. [11] have noted that when two shapes X and Y are related by a bijective correspondence $t : X \rightarrow Y$ and endowed with measures μ_X and μ_Y, then for any real function $f : X \rightarrow \mathbb{R}$, one can construct a corresponding function $g : Y \rightarrow \mathbb{R}$ as $g : f \circ t^{-1}$. In other words, the correspondence t uniquely defines a mapping between the two function spaces $F(X, \mathbb{R}) \rightarrow F(Y, \mathbb{R})$, where $F(X, \mathbb{R})$ denotes the space of real functions on X. Equipping X and Y with harmonic bases, $\{\phi_i\}_{i \geq 1}$ and $\{\psi_j\}_{j \geq 1}$, respectively, one can represent a function $f : X \rightarrow \mathbb{R}$ using the set of (generalized) Fourier coefficients $\{a_i\}_{i \geq 1}$ as $f = \sum_{i \geq 1} a_i \phi_i$.

Translating this representation into the other harmonic basis $\{\psi_j\}_{j \geq 1}$, one obtains a simple representation of the correspondence between the shapes given by $T(f) = \sum_{i,j \geq 1} a_i c_{ij} \psi_j$ where c_{ij} are Fourier coefficients of the basis functions of X expressed in the basis of Y, defined as $T(\phi_i) = \sum_{i,j \geq 1} c_{ij} \psi_j$. The correspondence t between the shapes can thus be approximated using k basis functions and encoded using a $k \times k$ matrix $C = (c_{ij})$ of these Fourier coefficients, referred to as the functional matrix. In this representation, the computation of the shape correspondence $t : X \rightarrow Y$ is translated into a simpler task of determining the functional matrix C from a set of correspondence constraints. The matrix C has a diagonal structure if the harmonic bases $\{\phi_i\}_{i \geq 1}$ and $\{\psi_j\}_{j \geq 1}$ are compatible, which is a crucial property for the efficient computation of the correspondence.

3.2   Analyzing Functional Maps

Here, the main goal is to isolate the regions where the map has induced significant distortion at various scales. This is simply achieved by considering the functional representation of a map C and performing spectral analysis on this representation, as shown in Figs. 1 and 2. It is expected that for an optimal map

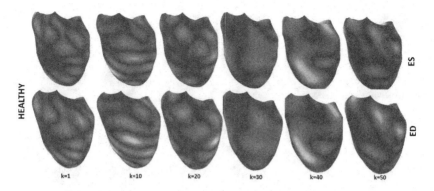

Fig. 1. The region where the map has distorted the area measure the most, at various scales k for an exemplary healthy subject. Note that the region is becoming more and more local with increasing values of k.

$t : X \rightarrow Y$, μ_X and μ_Y should be preserved. For the analysis and visualization of the distortion, Ovsjanikov et al. [12] and Rustamov et al. [13] proposed to use a real valued function $w : Y \rightarrow \mathbb{R}$ which will be used for mapping distortions on Y and $w \circ t$ for X. We have chosen area-distortion similar to [13] as the preferred measure of distortion.

It is proved in [12], that the optimal w can be derived by $w_k^* = \phi_{1...k}^N w$ where $\phi_{1...k}^N$ contains the first k eigenfunctions of the surface Laplacian operator and w is the right singular vector corresponding to the largest singular value of C. In addition, the scalars S_k has the ability to quantify the distortion at the various scales k. It is interesting to note that this technique does not place any assumptions on the geometry or topology of the function w, but provides a scale parameter k, which is more intuitive for understanding the scales of distortion. Large values of k allow for highly localized distortions, whereas medium and small values of k enforce the indicator functions to be more smooth resulting in the determination of globally problematic regions. In particular, the singular values C associated with each singular vector, indicates the amount of distortion introduced by the map at that particular scale.

3.3 Supervised Learning of Shape Distortions

We propose to learn the areas where the map has induced significant distortion between the End Systole and the End Diastole phases of a healthy versus diseased subject. In particular, we have achieved this by learning singular values associated with distortions at multiple scales concatenated with the difference of overall surface area of endo and epicardium at ES and ED. We subtracted the total area of endocardium at ED from the total are of endocardium at ES. We repeated the same operation for epicardium and used both features. We have chosen the vector of singular values $c_k \in C$ as the feature vector representing the distortion between ES and ED. The STACOM 2015 dataset contains labeled

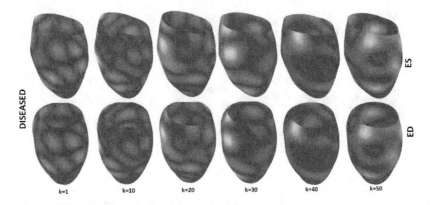

Fig. 2. The region where the map has distorted the area measure the most, at various scales k for an exemplary diseased subject.

dataset of 100 healthy and 100 diseased subjects, which is used for training a decision boundary of Support Vector Machine (SVM). During testing, similar feature selection procedure is used, followed by evaluation using the learnt decision boundary to consider whether the given meshes are from a normal subject or from a diseased one.

4   Implementation

We have employed a two step strategy for practical implementation of the problem, due to computational complexity of the method described in Sect. 3. In particular, we have adopted a Active Shape Model (ASM) [4] to resolve the relatively easier test cases. Eight different ASMs are trained on training datasets, four for normal and four for diseased cases. For either normal or diseased case, one ASM is trained for ES epi and endocardium, as well as ED epi and endocardium. For the test cases, the representative class of each surface is determined by finding the lower L_2 error across all points. The first screening of test cases results in determination of a class if 3 of the 4 shapes agree to a common class. Otherwise the test case is evaluated using the method described in Sect. 3.

We have used the *Mesh Laplacian* implementation of [15], for computing the basis functions. These basis functions are used for the functional map calculation and analysis. It is important to note that because of the orthonormality of our chosen basis, matrix of area-based inner product reduces to the identity matrix. Surface area of LV endo and epicardium meshes are calculated using the implementation of [6]. The supervised learning using SVM is performed using the *libSVM* implementation of Chang et al. [3]. In particular we have chosen a polynomial kernel of the following form $(\gamma u'v + c)^d$, where $\gamma = 2$, $c = 2$ and $d = 5$.

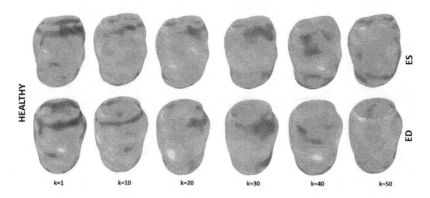

Fig. 3. The region where the map has distorted the area measure the most over the whole population of healthy subjects from STACOM 2015 training dataset, at various scales k.

5   Results

5.1   Data

Here we use the data available through the STACOM 2015 challenge for modeling the statistical shape of the left ventricle (LV). The STACOM training dataset contains 100 cases with myocardial infarction and another 100 healthy cases. The myocardial infarction cases are acquired through DETERMINE and the healthy ones through MESA [5]. In particular, the MESA study protocol ensured that these subjects did not have physician-diagnosed heart attack, angina, stroke, heart failure of atrial fibrillation, or undergone procedures related to cardiovascular disease. The testing set contains another set of 100 healthy and 100 diseased cases, for which the disease status is unknown to us and is evaluated by the co-organizers.

5.2   Qualitative Evaluation

To evaluate our preliminary results qualitatively, we have chosen to visualize the multi-scale distortion measure between ES and ED phases of a randomly sampled healthy and diseased subject as shown in Figs. 1 and 2. Since this yielded promising results, as evidenced from the multi-scale nature of the distortion, we have tried to further characterize population-level distortions between ES and ED phase of healthy and diseased subjects. In Figs. 3 and 4, population-level multiscale distortions of healthy and diseased subject respectively, are projected on two exemplary surfaces to visualize the differences. Different patterns of distortion is quite evident from Figs. 3 and 4, which motivates us for further quantitative analysis using machine learning techniques and check the accuracy of the proposed method in the STACOM 2015 challenge.

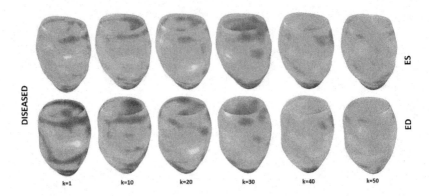

Fig. 4. The region where the map has distorted the area measure the most over the whole population of diseased subjects from STACOM 2015 training dataset, at various scales k.

5.3 Quantitative Evaluation

We have evaluated our algorithm on the training data set to estimate the performance. We have used a 10-fold cross-validation to evaluate the performance of the method and we have reached an average accuracy of 95.67 and a standard deviation of 1.26.

Furthermore, we have built a set-up to estimate the effect of number of training subjects on the accuracy. Figure 5 shows the influence of varying the total number of training subjects n, equally divided between normal and diseased cases, from $n = 20$ to $n = 180$ with the rest as testing subjects. The training samples are sampled randomly and for each n, we have run 50 experiments and reported the mean accuracy. It can be observed that increasing number of training subjects enable the algorithm to reach higher training accuracy.

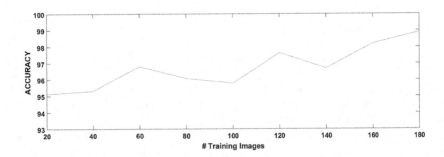

Fig. 5. The influence of the number of training subjects on accuracy

6 Discussions and Conclusion

Myocardial infarction results in a significant change of LV geometry due to the cardiac remodeling phenomenon. In this paper, we have proposed a framework to effectively differentiate the distortion between ES and ED phase of a healthy LV and diseased LV. Our proposed multi-scale approach is capable of describing distortions from global to local scale, which we have exploited in a supervised learning framework for the STACOM 2015 challenge. The preliminary visualizations and quantitative results suggest a population-wide common distortion pattern for healthy LVs, which can be utilized further in larger clinical studies. In this work, we have not considered the clinical quantities for describing cardiac remodeling such as Wall Thickness, Conicity, Sphericity etc. In the future, these quantities can be easily incorporated into the feature vector, to enhance the quantitative performance. Finally, the quantification of the distortion using singular values enable the possibility to extend this method for longitudinal studies of diseased LVs, and quantification of distortion over time.

References

1. Augenstein, K.F., et al.: Finite element modeling for three-dimensional motion reconstruction and analysis. In: Amini, A.A., Prince, J.L. (eds.) MCDM. Computational Imaging and Vision, vol. 23, pp. 37–58. Springer, The Netherlands (2001)
2. Bild, D.E., et al.: Multi-ethnic study of atherosclerosis: objectives and design. AJE **156**(9), 871–881 (2002)
3. Chang, C.C., et al.: LIBSVM: a library for support vector machines. TIST **2**(3), 27 (2011)
4. Cootes, T.F., et al.: Active shape models - their training and application. CVIU **61**(1), 38–59 (1995)
5. Fonseca, C.G., et al.: The cardiac atlas project-an imaging database for computational modeling and statistical atlases of the heart. Bioinformatics **27**(16), 2288–2295 (2011)
6. Legland, D.: Geom3d Toolbox. http://de.mathworks.com/matlabcentral/fileexchange/24484-geom3d
7. Li, B., et al.: In-line automated tracking for ventricular function with magnetic resonance imaging. JACC **3**(8), 860–866 (2010)
8. Mukhopadhyay, A., Qian, Z., Bhandarkar, S., Liu, T., Voros, S.: Shape analysis of the left ventricular endocardial surface and its application in detecting coronary artery disease. In: Metaxas, D.N., Axel, L. (eds.) FIMH 2011. LNCS, vol. 6666, pp. 275–283. Springer, Heidelberg (2011)
9. Mukhopadhyay, A., Qian, Z., Bhandarkar, S.M., Liu, T., Rinehart, S., Voros, S.: Morphological analysis of the left ventricular endocardial surface and its clinical implications. In: Ayache, N., Delingette, H., Golland, P., Mori, K. (eds.) MICCAI 2012, Part II. LNCS, vol. 7511, pp. 502–510. Springer, Heidelberg (2012)
10. Mukhopadhyay, A., et al.: Morphological analysis of the left ventricular endocardial surface using a bag-of-features descriptor. IEEE J-BHI **19**(4), 1483–1493 (2014)
11. Ovsjanikov, M., et al.: Functional maps: a flexible representation of maps between shapes. SIGGRAPH **31**(4), 30 (2012)

12. Ovsjanikov, M., et al.: Analysis and visualization of maps between shapes. CGF **32**(6), 135–145 (2013)

13. Rustamov, R.M., et al.: Map-based exploration of intrinsic shape differences and variability. ACM TOG **32**(4), 72 (2013)

14. Wong, S.P., et al.: Relation of left ventricular sphericity to 10-year survival after acute myocardial infarction. AJC **94**(10), 1270–1275 (2004)

15. Peyre, G.: Toolbox Graph. http://www.mathworks.com/matlabcentral/fileexchange/5355-toolbox-graph

Joint Clustering and Component Analysis of Spatio-Temporal Shape Patterns in Myocardial Infarction

Catarina Pinto[1]([✉]), Serkan Çimen[1], Ali Gooya[1],
Karim Lekadir[2], and Alejandro F. Frangi[1]

[1] Centre for Computational Imaging and Simulation
Technologies in Biomedicine (CISTIB),
University of Sheffield, Sheffield, UK
a.c.piuto@Sheffield.ac.uk, catarinapp24@gmail.com
[2] CISTIB, Universitat Pompeu Fabra, Barcelona, Spain

Abstract. The Left Ventricle (LV) undergoes remodelling after Myocardial Infarction (MI). In order to quantify the remodelling status, clinicians make use of conventional measures, not fully exploiting the available shape information. To characterize the changes in heart shape and classify heart data as normal or infarcted, we use a hierarchical generative model, which jointly clusters shape point sets from LV in End-Systolic (ED) and End-Systolic (ES) phases, and estimates the probability density function (pdf) of each cluster. We use a Variational Bayes (VB) method to infer the clusters labels, the mean models, and variation modes for the clusters. We also present the results in the supervised setting, where the labels of training data sets are given. Our classification results are evaluated in terms of sensitivity, specificity, and accuracy using 200 LV shapes provided by MICCAI 2015 STACOM LV Statistical Shape Modelling Challenge. Our method successfully classifies the data, achieving a specificity of 0.92 ± 0.06 and a sensitivity of 0.96 ± 0.07 for the supervised learning approach, and a specificity of 0.83 ± 0.03 and a sensitivity of 0.97 ± 0.01 for the unsupervised learning approach.

1   Introduction

Myocardial infarction may lead to the remodelling of the heart [3]. The increase in size and the sphericalization of the heart due to remodelling are usually linked to reduced life expectancy [16]. Clinical indices derived from mass and volume of the heart shape are employed to detect the remodelling and to assess the severity of it in current clinical practice. These conventional indices do not account for the heart shape or alterations of it during remodelling [16].

A detailed analysis of the shape of the heart could reveal information related to the status of the remodelling, since it contains more information compared to mass and volume. Specifically, a statistical analysis of the heart shapes from a population can yield new clinical indices derived from the variability of that population.

© Springer International Publishing Switzerland 2016
O. Camara et al. (Eds.): STACOM 2015, LNCS 9534, pp. 171–179, 2016.
DOI: 10.1007/978-3-319-28712-6_19

Statistical shape models (SSM) have been widely used in medical imaging, constituting robust tools for segmentation, recognition, and interpretation of real structures [4,6,9]. A SSM of the heart can have great importance since it allows to visualize shape differences, which are significant when comparing asymptomatic patients and patients whose heart shape has undergone remodelling [16].

Several studies have investigated the use of shape information to quantify the status of cardiac remodelling. Su *et al.* [14] assessed remodelling using curvature based shape descriptors extracted from 3D LV surface partitions. Normal and MI populations are compared via hypothesis testing.

Another popular way to exploit the shape information is to built a cardiac atlas and to study its variations [1,11,16]. These methods differ in terms of their strategy to compute the mean shape and deviations from it. Ardekani *et al.* [1] constructed a cardiac atlas and studied its variations to differentiate between ischemic and nonischemic cardiomyopathy patients. Average shapes of the LV for end diastole (ED) and end systole (ES) of each population were constructed using linear and non-linear registration techniques. Lamata *et al.* [11] applied SSM to investigate changes in the LV shapes of pregnant women with hypertension during pregnancy and with uncomplicated pregnancy. A LV template was fitted to manually segment slices and calculate the deviations from the template in both populations. Zhang *et al.* [16] built a statistical atlas to study the variations of LV shape after MI. Logistic regression was implemented using parameters that encode the variations to classify normal and remodelled hearts. In atlas based investigation of the LV shape, principal component analysis (PCA) is usually employed to analyse the variations in populations [1,11,16]. To this end, correspondences between the shapes must be established. Also, the knowledge of the labels can be either taken into account [1,11] or not [16]. In the first case, PCA is applied to normal and remodelled populations separately. In the latter, not accounting for label information ignores the possibility of having multi-model distributions for the shape population. In [16], PCA was applied to ED, ES and ED+ES shapes. It was concluded that ED+ES outperformed ED or ES alone and that the shape indices found characterized the data better than standard clinical measures.

In this paper, we aim to compute statistical models of the LV and detect the presence of MI. To accomplish this goal, we use a hierarchical generative model which jointly clusters the data and learns the pdf of each cluster. Our model is a flexible shape modelling approach which can work with correspondenceless point sets and can automatically identify the number of clusters. Although the model is originally devised for unsupervised learning of the pdfs of point sets, it can be adapted for supervised learning, given training data.

2   Method

In order to accomplish both the construction of a SSM and the classification of the left ventricular data, we used a hierarchical generative model [8]. Our model is structured in two layers that interact with each other and jointly estimates the underlying pdf of the point sets, constructs a SSM of the heart data, and clusters the point sets.

At the lower level, points sets are considered as samples from a Gaussian Mixture Model (GMM). This level is responsible for resampling the points sets and establishing correspondences between shapes. The means of the GMM are concatenated, constructing a higher dimensional vector in the higher level. This vector is regarded as a sample from a mixture of probabilistic principal component analyzers (PPCA), which is essentially a higher dimensional GMM. The clustering and linear component analysis take place in this level. An approximate inference algorithm based on a Variational Bayes (VB) method is utilized for unsupervised learning of clusters and their variations.

Let $\boldsymbol{\mathcal{X}}_k$ denote the kth point set ($1 \leq k \leq K$) represented by N_k points. Moreover, let x_{kn} denote the nth D-dimensional point of the kth point set. In the lower level, $\boldsymbol{\mathcal{X}}_k$ is considered to be consisted of the D-dimensional samples from an underlying GMM with M Gaussian components. The means are concatenated to a MD dimensional vector that represents $\boldsymbol{\mathcal{X}}_k$, being a resampled version of it.

In the higher level, the MD-dimensional vectors are assumed to be samples from a mixture of J PPCA. A PPCA is specified by its mean $\bar{\boldsymbol{\mu}}_j \in \mathbb{R}^{MD}$ and the subspace component of the covariance matrix in the form $\boldsymbol{W}_j\boldsymbol{W}_j^T$. The projection of $\boldsymbol{\mathcal{X}}_k$ onto the space spanned by principal components of the jth cluster is given by

$$\mu_{jk} = \boldsymbol{W}_j\boldsymbol{v}_k + \bar{\boldsymbol{\mu}}_j \tag{1}$$

where $\boldsymbol{v}_k$ are the loading coefficients. This equation describes the interaction between both layers.

The latent variables, $\boldsymbol{\theta}$, are identified as the membership vectors for both levels of the GMM, principal component matrices, loading vectors and variance of the PPCAs (see [6] for details). The goal is to find the probability of the latent variables given the observed data, $p(\boldsymbol{\theta}|\boldsymbol{\mathcal{X}})$, which is intractable. Instead, we aim to approximate it with an another distribution $q(\boldsymbol{\theta})$, which is assumed to be factorizable w.r.t. disjoint groups of the latent variables.

The Kullback-Leibler (KL) divergence between the real distribution $p(\boldsymbol{\theta}|\boldsymbol{\mathcal{X}})$ and the approximated posterior $q(\boldsymbol{\theta})$ should be minimized in order to estimate the latter. In practice, this is not feasible as the true posterior is not known. To overcome this, the Lower Bound (LB) is maximized, which is equivalent to minimizing KL.

The logarithm of the marginal probability, $ln(p(\boldsymbol{\mathcal{X}}))$, is a combination of the LB and the KL divergence:

$$ln(p(\boldsymbol{\mathcal{X}})) = LB(q(\boldsymbol{\theta})) + KL(p(\boldsymbol{\theta}|\boldsymbol{\mathcal{X}})||q(\boldsymbol{\theta})) \tag{2}$$

where,

$$LB = \int q(\boldsymbol{\theta}) \, ln \, \frac{p(\boldsymbol{\mathcal{X}}, \boldsymbol{\theta})}{q(\boldsymbol{\theta})} d\boldsymbol{\theta} \tag{3}$$

The maximum of the LB occurs when the KL divergence vanishes, i.e., when $q(\boldsymbol{\theta})$ equals the posterior distribution $p(\boldsymbol{\theta}|\boldsymbol{\mathcal{X}})$. One can develop further this formula until concluding that the logarithm of the optimal solution for one of the factors of $q(\boldsymbol{\theta})$ can be obtained from the logarithm of the joint distribution over all variables and then taking the expectation w.r.t. all of the other factors:

$$ln\, q_j^*(\boldsymbol{\theta}_j) = \mathbb{E}_{\theta\backslash\theta_j}\left[ln(p(\boldsymbol{\mathcal{X}},\boldsymbol{\theta}))\right] + const. \tag{4}$$

The set of above equations for all values of j represent a set of consistency conditions for the maximum of LB. As they depend on the expectation w.r.t other factors, they do not constitute an explicit solution. Therefore, finding the optimal approximate distribution is based on a iterative VB method: first all factors are initialized and then cycled over, being updated given the current estimation on the others, until convergence. In the end, both an approximation of the posterior probability of the unobserved variables, given the data, and a LB for the evidence $ln(p(\boldsymbol{\mathcal{X}}))$ are computed.

Although our method offers an unsupervised learning of point set clusters and their variations, it is easy to adapt it to supervised learning when training data is available. Specifically, in the unsupervised strategy we use the point sets without label information and compute mean models, variations and classification of the data from the estimated pdf. In the supervised strategy, we learn the mean models and variations given the labelled data and apply them to test data in order to only find the classification.

3   Experiments

Our method is evaluated using the LV dataset provided by MICCAI 2015 STA-COM Workshop LV Statistical Shape Modelling Challenge [5]. This dataset consisted of one hundred symptomatic and one hundred asymptomatic cases from DETERMINE [10] and MESA [2] datasets, respectively. Each shape comprises point sets at two cardiac phases: ED and ES.

The proposed method requires spatial alignment of LV shapes. The spatial alignment could either be incorporated into the formulation and estimated with other latent variables [7] or could be performed as a preprocessing step. This paper adopts the latter strategy to reduce computational complexity of the algorithm. Coherent Point Drift (CPD) [12] algorithm was selected for this task, since it offers a robust technique for the point set registration problem. This method interprets the alignment of two point sets as a probabilistic problem, while preserving the topological structure of the shapes. We opted for a similarity transformation to register point sets. The shapes were normalized to zero mean and unit variance prior to the registration process.

To achieve a non-biased registration, a mean ED model is computed by applying CPD registration to 10 normal and 10 infarcted LV shapes, which are selected randomly from those populations. Then, the 200 ED point sets are registered to that mean model. The transformation computed for each ED data is applied to the corresponding ES data from the same patient, to maintain consistency.

This is possible by assuming movement artefacts between the distinct capturing moments (ED and ES) present, if any, are minimal.

We perform both unsupervised and supervised learning in order to compute the mean models and classify the data, using a combination of ED and ES. By concatenating ED and ES data into a 6 dimensional matrix and applying our method, we can recover the data from ED and ES independently in the end of the process and construct mean models and variations for each case.

Different model parameters were tested in both approaches. The number of clusters (J) was set to 2, as there are 2 classes only: normal and infarcted LV. To find the optimal combination of the number of Gaussians of the GMM (M) and modes of variation (L), several experiments were conducted. Specifically, we searched for optimal values on a discrete grid of values varying between 300 to 1100, with increments of 100, and 1 to 4 for M and L, respectively. For the unsupervised learning, 4 experiments were repeated to each set of M-L combinations, in order to reduce the randomness resulting from the initialization algorithm. For the supervised learning, the M-L combinations were tested with leave-20-out cross-validation experiments. Specifically, in this approach we fixed M to the optimal value obtained for unsupervised learning and searched for optimal L value. We chose the M-L values that led to the highest LB value for each approach. In both supervised and unsupervised approaches, the results pointed to the same values for M and L (M = 1100, L = 3).

4 Results

4.1 Mean Models and Modes of Variation

Within each approach, 4 mean shapes were computed: ED Normal, ES Normal, ED Infarcted and ES Infarcted, which allows to compare not only infarcted to normal models but also to evaluate how important is the mode of contraction of the heart in each class.

Figure 1 shows the mean models resulting from the supervised approach and from the unsupervised approach. We can notice that the shapes from the supervised and unsupervised approaches resemble each other, which indicates the results from the unsupervised method are close to the ones created knowing *a priori* the class labels.

From the coronal and axial sections present in Fig. 2 one can see in more depth some details. The normal and infarcted shapes are quite distinct in terms of LV wall thickness and end systolic volume in the ES models, indicating that the contraction is stronger in normal hearts. Also, specifically in the ED model one can note that the normal mean shape is longer and less spherical than the infarcted one, which is supported by the literature [16].

Three modes of variation were computed for each mean shape. Figure 3 shows the modes of variations for the ED Normal shape, as an example. These modes of variation are associated with the elongation of the heart and the mitral valve orientation, for instance. Due to the isotropic noise model, W_j does not fully

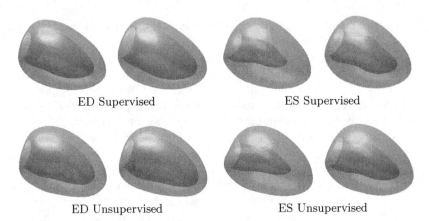

ED Supervised   ES Supervised

ED Unsupervised   ES Unsupervised

Fig. 1. The 4 mean models resulting from: supervised (top) and unsupervised (bottom) learning approaches. In each row, we have from left to right: ED Normal, ED Infarcted, ES Normal and ES Infarcted mean shapes.

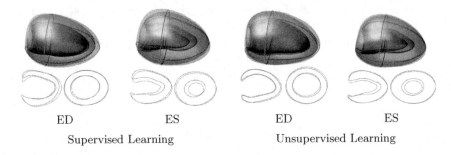

ED   ES   ED   ES
    Supervised Learning   Unsupervised Learning

Fig. 2. Comparision between normal and infarcted shapes: mean models (top) and axial and coronal cross sections (bottom), from supervised and unsupervised learning approaches. The normal and infarcted shapes are demonstrated in red and green color, respectively (Color figure online).

describe the variance and therefore the relationship between the loading coefficients v_k and the variance is not straightforward as in PCA [15].

4.2 Classification Results

In order to perform classification, we selected the M-L combination that led to the higher LB value. Table 1 shows some of the results for the supervised cross-validation tests, while in Table 2 one can see the unsupervised experiments results described in Sect. 3. It is possible to notice that the combination of $M = 1100$ and $L = 3$ has the highest LB value, while classifying successfully most of the data.

The results with higher LB achieved by our model have usually high sensitivity values as well (above 0.90 in this case). In the unsupervised tests performed with the optimal M-L combination, an average of 10 % of the data was incorrectly

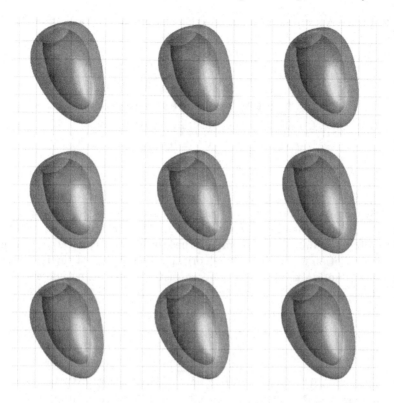

Fig. 3. Three modes of variation obtained for normal population at ED. Each row corresponds one mode of variation. In the middle column is the mean model and in the left and right are the variations from the mean computed by our method.

Table 1. Supervised results for the selection of Optimal L Parameter for M=1100

	Supervised		
	LB	Specificity	Sensitivity
L = 1	-2.105e+07	0.89 ± 0.10	0.93 ± 0.10
L = 2	-2.102e+07	0.88 ± 0.08	0.97 ± 0.07
L = 3	-2.102e+07	0.92 ± 0.06	0.96 ± 0.07
L = 4	-2.103e+07	0.92 ± 0.06	0.92 ± 0.08

classified. A specificity of 0.83 ± 0.03 and sensitivity of 0.97 ± 0.01 was achieved, as stated in Table 3. In the same table one can notice that high values of specificity (0.92 ± 0.06) and sensitivity (0.96 ± 0.07) were also achieved for the supervised approach. Therefore, both the unsupervised and the supervised approach show high classification accuracy (around 0.90, as seen in Table 3).

During the tests we concluded that the best LB value does not have a direct relation with best classification results. This shows the difference between

Table 2. Unsupervised results for the selection of Optimal L Parameter for M=1100

	Unsupervised		
	LB	Specificity	Sensitivity
L = 1	-2.352e+07	0.83 ± 0.03	0.96 ± 0.01
L = 2	-2.349e+07	0.85 ± 0.02	0.94 ± 0.03
L = 3	-2.348e+07	0.83 ± 0.03	0.97 ± 0.01
L = 4	-2.349e+07	0.85 ± 0.02	0.95 ± 0.01

explaining and predicting about data: the method that best explains, i.e. with higher LB, not always predicts the best [13]. Also, we stated that the initialization has influence on the performance of the classification. Specifically, the amount and type of data used to compute the initialization can lead to a decrease of the generalization capacity of the algorithm. The quality of the initialization is, therefore, important and should be consistent when using supervised and unsupervised methods.

Table 3. Classification results

	Specificity	Sensitivity	Accuracy
Supervised (M = 1100, L = 3)	0.91 ± 0.06	0.97 ± 0.07	0.94 ± 0.06
Unsupervised (M = 1100, L = 3)	0.83 ± 0.03	0.97 ± 0.01	0.90 ± 0.02

5   Conclusion

In brief, we use a hierarchical generative model that clusters the point sets into normal and infarcted hearts, finding also the mean models and intra-clusters variations. 4 mean shape models were constructed: ED Normal, ED Infarcted, ES Normal and ES Infarcted. That was accomplished by joining the ED and ES data from the same patient into a 6 dimensional matrix, running our method and then independently analysing ED and ES. 3 modes of variation were computed for each model. The classification results of the data into normal and infarcted presented high specificity and sensitivity values, specifically when choosing model parameters that had correspondent high LB values.

The computed mean models are in accordance with the literature, as it is visually possible to notice a longer and less spherical shape in the normal mean heart (see Fig. 2). Also, differences in wall thickness from ED to ES were spotted, specially in the infarcted shapes.

The major contribution of the paper lies in the fact that the shape information can be used by clinicians to diagnose and evaluate MI, as stated before in [16].

We prove that our method successfully and accurately clusters the data and distinguishes between normal and infarcted hearts, while also capturing the mean shape and intra-class variation, both in the supervised and unsupervised approach.

References

1. Ardekani, S., Weiss, R.G., Lardo, A.C., George, R.T., Lima, J.A.C., Wu, K.C., Miller, M.I., Winslow, R.L., Younes, L.: Computational method for identifying and quantifying shape features of human left ventricular remodeling. Ann. Biomed. Eng. **37**(6), 1043–1054 (2009)
2. Bild, D., Bluemke, D., Burke, G., Detrano, R., Roux, A., et al.: Multi-ethnic study of atherosclerosis: objectives and design. Am. J. Epidemiol. **156**, 871–881 (2002)
3. Cohn, J.N., Ferrari, R., Sharpe, N.: Cardiac remodeling-concepts and clinical implications: a consensus paper from an international forum on cardiac remodeling. J. Am. Coll. Cardiol. **35**(3), 569–582 (2000)
4. Cootes, T., Taylor, C.: Statistical models of appearance for medical image analysis and computer vision. Proc. SPIE Med. Imaging **4322**, 236–248 (2001)
5. Fonseca, C.G., Backhaus, M., Bluemke, D.A., Britten, R.D., Do Chung, J., Cowan, B.R., Young, A.A., Do Chung, J., Cowan, B.R., Young, A.A.: The cardiac atlas project–an imaging database for computational modeling and statistical atlases of the heart. Bioinformatics **27**(16), 2288–2295 (2011)
6. Frangi, A.F., Rueckert, D., Schnabel, J.A., Niessen, W.J.: Automatic construction of multiple-object three-dimensional statistical shape models: Application to cardiac modeling. IEEE Trans. Med. Imaging **21**, 1151–1166 (2002)
7. Gooya, A., Davatzikos, C., Frangi, A.F.: A bayesian approach to sparse model selection in statistical shape models. SIAM J. Imaging Sci. **8**(2), 858–887 (2015)
8. Gooya, A., Lekadir, K., Alba, X., Swift, A.J., Wild, J.M., Frangi, A.F.: Joint clustering and component analysis of correspondenceless point sets: application to cardiac statistical modeling. In: Ourselin, S., Alexander, D.C., Westin, C.-F., Cardoso, M.J. (eds.) IPMI 2015. LNCS, vol. 9123, pp. 98–109. Springer, Heidelberg (2015)
9. Heimann, T., Meinzer, H.P.: Statistical shape models for 3D medical image segmentation: a review. Med. Image Anal. **13**(4), 543–563 (2009)
10. Kadish, A., Bello, D., Finn, J., Bonow, R., Schaechter, A., et al.: Rationale and design for the defibrillators to reduce risk by magnetic resonance imaging evaluation (determine) trial. J. Cardiovasc. Electrophysiol. **20**, 982–987 (2009)
11. Lamata, P., Lazdam, M., Ashcroft, A., Lewandowski, A.J., Leeson, P., Smith, N.: Computational mesh as a descriptor of left ventricular shape for clinical diagnosis. Comput. Cardiol. **40**, 571–574 (2013)
12. Myronenko, A., Song, X.: Point set registration: coherent point drift. IEEE PAMI **32**(12), 1–14 (2010)
13. Shmueli, G.: To explain or to predict? Stat. Sci. **25**(3), 289–310 (2010)
14. Su, Y., Zhong, L., Lim, C.W., Ghista, D., Chua, T., Tan, R.S.: A geometrical approach for evaluating left ventricular remodeling in myocardial infarct patients. Comput. Methods Programs Biomed. **108**(2), 500–510 (2012)
15. Tipping, M., Bishop, C.: Mixtures of probabilistic principal component analyzers. Neural Comput. **11**(2), 443–482 (1999)
16. Zhang, X., Cowan, B.R., Bluemke, D.A., Finn, J.P., Fonseca, C.G., Kadish, A.H., Lee, D.C., Lima, J.A.C., Suinesiaputra, A., Young, A.A., Medrano-Gracia, P.: Atlas-based quantification of cardiac remodeling due to myocardial infarction. PLoS ONE **9**(10), e110243 (2014)

Myocardial Infarction Detection from Left Ventricular Shapes Using a Random Forest

Jack Allen[1(✉)], Ernesto Zacur[2], Erica Dall'Armellina[1], Pablo Lamata[2], and Vicente Grau[1]

[1] University of Oxford, Oxford, UK
jack.allen@jesus.ox.ac.uk
[2] King's College London, London, UK

Abstract. Understanding myocardial remodelling, and developing tools for its accurate quantification, is fundamental for improving the diagnosis and treatment of myocardial infarction patients. Conventional clinical metrics, such as blood pool volume or ejection fraction, are not always distinctive. Here we describe a method for the classification of myocardial infarction from 3D diastolic and systolic left ventricle shapes, represented by point sets. Classification features included global geometric, shape and thickness descriptors, and a random forest was used for classification. Results from cross validation show an accuracy of 92.5 % (leave-one-out) and 91.5 % (5-fold), improving the 87 % obtained with ejection fraction thresholds. These results suggest that refined remodelling metrics provide information beyond standard clinical descriptors.

Keywords: Statistical shape model · Random forest · Left ventricle · Myocardial infarction

1 Introduction

The damage resulting from myocardial infarction can cause the heart to remodel, which can have a negative effect on its function [13]. Remodelling of the left ventricle (LV) is particularly significant because of its potential life-threatening effects, and is currently characterised through global metrics, such as blood pool volume or LV ejection fraction. In particular, myocardial infarction can cause thinning and a decrease in thickness change over the cardiac cycle, in the area of the scar, while hypertrophy can occur in other areas as they adapt to compensate [13], and these are features not fully captured by current clinical metrics.

Shape and cardiac remodelling can also be characterised through statistical shape models, also known as computational statistical atlases [4,15]. To further the work of cardiac atlas research, schemes such as the Cardiac Atlas Project (CAP) have been set up. The CAP facilitates the sharing of software and data between investigators, across different institutions [5]. Atlas-based metrics have

---

The original version of this chapter was revised.
An erratum to this chapter can be found at 10.1007/978-3-319-28712-6_24.

© Springer International Publishing Switzerland 2016
O. Camara et al. (Eds.): STACOM 2015, LNCS 9534, pp. 180–189, 2016.
DOI: 10.1007/978-3-319-28712-6_20

the potential to increase specificity and sensitivity, and to improve our under-standing of shape changes in development and pathology [7,8]. In this work we explore this hypothesis, generating a large collection of LV shape metrics, and analysing its joint classification performance through Breiman's decision tree ensembles, known as *random forests* [3], a technique that has been shown to provide excellent classification results when many features are available. The objective is to provide metrics that capture the detailed anatomical changes caused by infarction.

2   Materials and Methods

2.1   The Data

A dataset of 400 3D left ventricle shapes was provided by the organisers of the MICCAI 2015 Statistical Atlases and Computational Modelling of the heart (STACOM) workshop. The shapes were from a large cardiac imaging database, built by the CAP. Each case included end-diastolic (ED) and end-systolic (ES) point coordinates (1089 points) and indices of triangle vertices previously fitted to magnetic resonance images as described in [16], with a correction for potential bias from different acquisition protocols [10]. For each of the cases, the indices of points approximately in the middle of the septum were also provided. Of the 400 shapes, 200 were labelled for use as training data. Of the training data, 100 were cases with myocardial infarction, from the DETERMINE trial [6]. The remaining 100 training cases were from the MESA study [2], where those enrolled did not show symptoms of myocardial infarction (these two cohorts will be referred to as DETERMINE and MESA, respectively). The remaining 200 unlabelled cases were used as an evaluation cohort by the challenge organisers, for which the results were submitted as an entry to the challenge.

2.2   Feature Computation

We calculated a combination of standard clinical features and novel atlas-based metrics, as described next (full list in Table 1). All metrics were computed using *MATLAB* and *The Visualization Tookit* (VTK) [12].

Volumes and Ejection Fraction. We calculated the volumes contained by the epicardium and endocardium surfaces, both at ED and ES. For this purpose, we closed each endocardial and epicardial surface by adding a node at the centroid of the boundary of the base and connecting this new node by a fan of triangles to the boundary. Once the surfaces were closed (and consistent normals pointing outwards were assigned to each triangle) we computed the volume within each surface, making use of the divergence theorem and integrating the flow through the surfaces [11]. These volumes were used to compute ejection fractions.

Sphericity. Remodelling has been shown to produce increased sphericity of the left ventricle [13]. We computed the sphericity [14] of the endocardium and epicardium surfaces at ED and ES using Eq. 1, where V and A are the volume and surface area of a 3D shape, respectively.

$$Sphericity = \frac{\pi^{1/3}(6V)^{2/3}}{A} \qquad (1)$$

Atlas-Based Shape Metrics. A statistical shape model, represented by a point distribution model, was built in a similar way to previous publications [1,9]. The 200 training cases were used to build the model. A mean shape $\bar{x}$ was computed by means of Procrustes iterations, without reflection or scaling components. Principal component analysis (PCA) was then applied to the training shapes, to find a matrix of eigenvectors Φ, with corresponding eigenvalues, describing geometric modes of variation across the shapes. After ranking the eigenvectors in descending order according to their corresponding eigenvalues, the first 100 were used in Eq. 2, to obtain atlas-based shape metrics b for each shape vector x. The eigenvalues describe the variance of the analysed population in terms of the corresponding eigenvector. This means that modes with relatively large eigenvalues will be comparatively more useful for separating two classes. With this in mind, we predicted that the first 100 modes would be sufficient for providing enough useful information for classification and that including modes with smaller variances would be unnecessary.

$$\mathbf{b} = \Phi^T(\mathbf{x} - \bar{\mathbf{x}}) \qquad (2)$$

Myocardium Thicknesses. We calculated the myocardium thicknesses for all the cases, at ES and ED. This was done by computing the distance between each node on the epicardium mesh and the closest point (not necessarily a node) on the endocardium surface. The shapes were divided into three segments, named: apical, middle and basal. Each segment consisted of an equal number of nodes in the long axis direction. Thickness statistics were computed for the whole left ventricle and each of these sections.

Atlas-Based Thickness Metrics. We also computed a statistical shape model of the thickness of the 100 training cases. Modes of thickness were found in a similar way to those of shape (i.e. using Eq. 2), but by applying PCA only on the MESA shapes, with the aim of making the model independent from the location of the scar within the ventricle, as well as the variability of the remodelling responses.

2.3   Classification

Random forests are ensembles of many decision trees built iteratively. To produce each tree, a subset of the cases, of predefined size, is randomly chosen (*i.e.* 'bagged') to be used for training. At an initial node, a subset of the features is randomly chosen and the feature that provides the optimal split is identified and used to divide the training data into two branches, to two new nodes. In our study, branches were produced until each new node only contained one class. Unused cases (*i.e.* 'out-of-bag' cases), were passed down each completed tree, and the most common prediction for each case was compared with the true label. The forest provided the probability (between 0 and 1) that each case belonged to either of the two classes. Each case was assigned the label of the class with a probability greater than a threshold (0.5).

Classification error was obtained by cross-validation, using 'k-fold' techniques with k = 5 and k = 200 (equivalent to a 'leave-one-out'). We used 300 trees in the ensemble, as this was sufficient for achieving error convergence. Fewer trees could possibly be used without significantly increasing the overall error. The 'out-of-bag' importance of each feature for successful classification was found individually, by randomly mixing the feature values, before passing the 'out-of-bag' cases down the tree again. The importance of each feature was the average increase in classification error caused by the mixing, for the whole ensemble, divided by the standard deviation.

The most relevant shape and thickness atlas metrics were selected according to their out-of-bag importance: the first 15 modes were chosen as features to build the final random forest. The features in Table 1 were also used to classify the test data as an entry to the challenge. The parameters for shape and thickness variation in the test shapes were produced by fitting the test shapes to the training data models.

3   Results

3.1   Classification

Ejection fraction was used to define a baseline for the classification performance in a conventional clinical setting, reporting an accuracy of 87 % (provided by two different thresholds as seen in Fig. 1). This result was improved to 92.5 % using the proposed classification strategy, as reported in Fig. 4. This result was achieved after the selection of atlas-based features guided by the out-of-bag importance illustrated in Fig. 2. Figure 5 compares the random forest ROC curve, with that of the ejection fractions, and it is clear that the random forest ROC curve covers a larger area. Rounded to two decimal places, the areas under the random forest and ejection fraction curves were 0.98 and 0.94, respectively. There was also an improvement in the specificity associated with the optimal accuracy (94 % and 83 %, to 97 %). The random forest ROC curve was obtained by varying the threshold applied to the probability of the DETERMINE class, from 0 to 1. For each threshold value, all the 'out-of-bag' training cases were classified. For example, when the threshold was 0, all of the cases were assigned the label of DETERMINE. Figure 3 shows the importance of the complete list of features (described in Table 1), and reveals that the relative importance of the atlas-based metrics changed. The most relevant mode of shape variation is

Table 1. The complete list of features used for classification.

Index	Feature
1	Ejection fraction
2:16	Shape model parameters for modes 1:15
17:20	Sphericity (endocardium and epicardium at ED and ES)
21:22	Mean thickness (ED and ES)
23	Absolute difference in mean thickness between ED and ES
24:25	Mode thickness (ED and ES)
26:27	Median thickness (ED and ES)
28:29	Thickness variance (ED and ES)
30	Thickness difference variance
31	Thickness variance (ED with ES)
32:34	Segment thickness variance (ED: apical, middle and basal)
35:37	Segment thickness variance (ES: apical, middle and basal)
38:40	Segment thickness variance (ED with ES: apical, middle and basal)
41:43	Segment thickness mean (ED: apical, middle and basal)
44:46	Segment thickness mean (ES: apical, middle and basal)
47:49	Segment thickness mean (ED with ES: apical, middle and basal)
50:51	Volumes (ES endocardium and epicardium)
52:53	Volumes (ED endocardium and epicardium)
54:55	Log volumes (ES endocardium and epicardium)
56:57	Log volumes (ED endocardium and epicardium)
58:72	Thickness model parameters for modes 1:15

illustrated in Fig. 6, where a variation in thickness can be seen at the apex at ED, and changes in endocardium curvature, particularly opposite the middle of the septum, can be seen at ES.

4 Discussion

As expected according to clinical practice, ejection fraction proved to be a robust marker (87 % accuracy). Additional features improved the classification of infarct and control subjects, reaching a cross-validated accuracy of 92.5 %. Although the random forest ROC curve in Fig. 5 was not produced with k-fold cross-validation (used for the classification errors in Fig. 4), Fig. 5 suggests that an improvement in performance was achieved by the random forest.

In the search for the most relevant classification markers, our results revealed that ES endocardium volume is slightly more important than ejection fraction (Fig. 3). Despite both measures being strongly correlated, they still revealed a large complementary value. The third metric that contributed to the decisions in

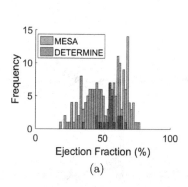
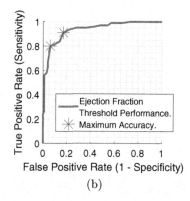

Fig. 1. 1(a) Comparing the ejection fractions of the DETERMINE and MESA cases 1(b) Ejection fraction ROC curve. Red stars mark the sensitivity (80 % and 91 %) and specificity (94 % and 83 %) values for the maximum accuracy achieved (87 %) when thresholds were applied to the ejection fractions alone (Color figure online).

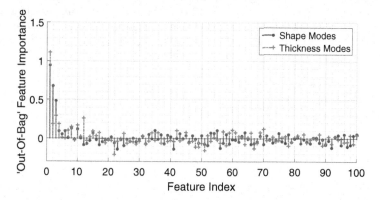

Fig. 2. Importance of the first 100 modes of variation of the two models.

our classifier was the variance in the thickness difference between ED and ES, a surrogate of the heterogeneity of contraction (infarcted cases will have a reduced contraction in scarred areas). Relatively, the atlas-based metrics made a small contribution to the classification. The analysis revealed additional insights about the remodelling pattern in infarction, with changes in endocardial curvature and apical thickness detected (see Fig. 6). Perhaps these areas of the ventricle were common sites of infarction within the training cases.

The selection of atlas-based metrics was made in a preliminary stage (see Fig. 2), but results revealed that this may have led to a sub-optimal result: the importance of particular shape and thickness atlas metrics increased when used along with the remaining features in Table 1 (e.g. shape mode 14 and thickness mode 7). This suggests that these modes provide different information to the ejection fraction and volumes measurements, and could represent an interesting

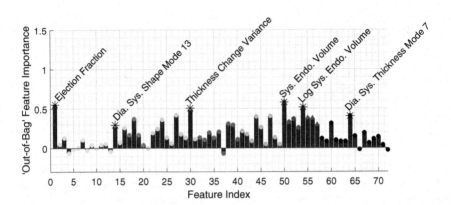

Fig. 3. Random forest importance of all the features specified in Table 1. The colours group the features according to Table 1. (yellow = shape model parameters, magenta = sphericity, cyan = global thickness statistics, red = segment thickness variances, green = segment thickness means, blue circles = volumes, blue triangles = log volumes, black = thickness model parameters) (Color figure online).

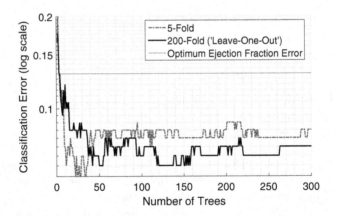

Fig. 4. Cross-validated (5-fold and leave-one-out) classification error for the random forest built using all the features listed in Table 1.

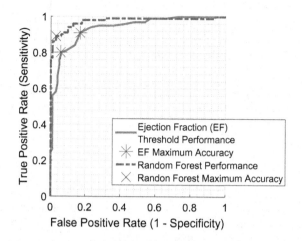

Fig. 5. Comparison of the ROC curve for the final random forest, with that of the ejection fractions already shown in Fig. 1(b). The data for these curves were collated without any cross-validation. True positive rate is also known as specificity. Red stars mark the sensitivity (80 % and 91 %) and specificity (94 % and 83 %) values for the maximum accuracy achieved (87 %) when thresholds were applied to the ejection fractions alone. The green cross marks the sensitivity (89 %) and specificity (97 %) associated with the maximum accuracy for the random forest ROC curve (93 %) (Color figure online).

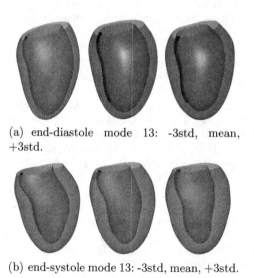

(a) end-diastole mode 13: -3std, mean, +3std.

(b) end-systole mode 13: -3std, mean, +3std.

Fig. 6. Variation for the statistical shape model mode with the highest importance when used with all other features. The points approximately in line with the middle of the septum are shown in black.

avenue for future research. The use of a random forest allowed us to identify these complementary sources of discriminative information, but further work is needed to find the optimal list of anatomical features, in terms of both the classification performance and the number of features used.

Acknowledgements. This work was supported by funding from the Medical Research Council (MRC) and Engineering and Physical Sciences Research Council (EPSRC) [grant number EP/L016052/1].

References

1. van Assen, H.C., Danilouchkine, M.G., Frangi, A.F., Ordas, S., Westenberg, J.J., Reiber, J.H., Lelieveldt, B.P.: SPASM: a 3D-ASM for segmentation of sparse and arbitrarily oriented cardiac MRI data. Med. Image Anal. **10**(2), 286–303 (2006). http://www.ncbi.nlm.nih.gov/pubmed/16439182

2. Bild, D.E., Bluemke, D.A., Burke, G.L., Detrano, R., Diez Roux, A.V., Folsom, A.R., Greenland, P., Jacobs Jr., D.R., Kronmal, R., Liu, K., Nelson, J.C., OLeary, D., Saad, M.F., Shea, S., Szklo, M., Tracy, R.P.: Multi-ethnic study of atherosclerosis: objectives and design. Am. J. Epidemiol. **156**(9), 871–881 (2002). http://aje.oxfordjournals.org/content/156/9/871.abstract

3. Breiman, L.: Random forests. Mach. Learn. **45**(1), 5–32 (2001). http://link.springer.com/article/10.1023/A:1010933404324

4. Cootes, T.F., Cooper, D.H., Taylor, C.J., Graham, J.: Trainable method of parametric shape description. Image Vis. Comput. **10**(5), 289–294 (1992). http://www.sciencedirect.com/science/article/pii/0262885692900444

5. Fonseca, C.G., Backhaus, M., Bluemke, D.A., Britten, R.D., Chung, J.D., Cowan, B.R., Dinov, I.D., Finn, J.P., Hunter, P.J., Kadish, A.H., Lee, D.C., Lima, J.A.C., MedranoGracia, P., Shivkumar, K., Suinesiaputra, A., Tao, W., Young, A.A.: The Cardiac Atlas Project - an imaging database for computational modeling and statistical atlases of the heart. Bioinformatics **27**(16), 2288–2295 (2011). http://bioinformatics.oxfordjournals.org/content/27/16/2288.abstract

6. Kadish, A.H., Bello, D., Finn, P., Bonow, R.O., Schaechter, A., Subacius, H., Albert, C., Daubert, J.P., Fonseca, C., Goldberger, J.J.: Rationale and design for the defibrillators to reduce risk by magnetic resonance imaging evaluation (determine) trial. J. Cardiovasc. Electrophysiol. **20**(9), 982–987 (2009). http://www.ncbi.nlm.nih.gov/pmc/articles/PMC3128996/

7. Lewandowski, A.J., Augustine, D., Lamata, P., Davis, E.F., Lazdam, M., Francis, J., McCormick, K., Wilkinson, A., Singhal, A., Lucas, A., Smith, N., Neubauer, S., Leeson, P.: The preterm heart in adult life: cardiovascular magnetic resonance reveals distinct differences in left ventricular mass, geometry and function. Circulation **127**(2), 197–206 (2012). http://dx.doi.org/10.1161/circulationaha.112.126920

8. Lorenz, C., Berg, J.V.: A comprehensive shape model of the heart. Med. Image Anal. **10**(4), 657–670 (2006)

9. Lötjönen, J., Kivistö, S., Koikkalainen, J., Smutek, D., Lauerma, K.: Statistical shape model of atria, ventricles and epicardium from short- and long-axis MR images. Med. Image Anal. **8**(3), 371–386 (2004)

10. Medrano-Gracia, P., Cowan, B.R., Bluemke, D.A., Finn, J.P., Kadish, A.H., Lee, D.C., Lima, J.A.C., Suinesiaputra, A., Young, A.A.: Atlas-based analysis of cardiac shape and function correction of regional shape bias due to imaging protocol for population studies. J. Cardiovasc. Magn. Reson (official journal of the Society for Cardiovascular Magnetic Resonance) 15, 80 (2013). ISBN:1097-6647

11. Millán, R.D., Dempere-Marco, L., Pozo, J.M., Cebral, J.R., Frangi, F.: Morphological characterization of intracranial aneurysms using 3-D moment invariants. IEEE Trans. Med. Imaging 26(9), 1270–1282 (2007)

12. Schroeder, W., Martin, K., Lorensen, B.: The Visualization Toolkit, 4th edn. Kitware Inc., Clifton Park (2006)

13. Sutton, M.G.S.J., Sharpe, N.: Left ventricular remodeling after myocardial infarction: pathophysiology and therapy. Circulation 101(25), 2981–2988 (2000). http://circ.ahajournals.org/content/101/25/2981.short

14. Wadell, H.: Sphericity and roundness of rock particles. J. Geol. 41(3), 310–331 (1933)

15. Young, A.A., Frangi, A.F.: Computational cardiac atlases: from patient to population and back. Exp. Physiol. 94(5), 578–596 (2009). http://www.ncbi. nlm.nih.gov/pubmed/19098087

16. Young, A.A., Cowan, B.R., Thrupp, S.F., Hedley, W.J., DellItalia, L.J.: Left ventricular mass and volume: fast calculation with guide-point modeling on MR images. Radiology 216(2), 597–602 (2000). http://pubs.rsna.org/doi/abs/ 10.1148/radiology.216.2.r00au14597

Combination of Polyaffine Transformations and Supervised Learning for the Automatic Diagnosis of LV Infarct

Marc-Michel Rohé[✉], Nicolas Duchateau, Maxime Sermesant,
and Xavier Pennec

Inria Sophia-Antipolis, Asclepios Research Group, Sophia-Antipolis, France
marc-michel.rohe@inria.fr

Abstract. In this article, we present an application of the polyaffine transformations to classify a population of hearts with myocardial infarction. Polyaffine transformations aim at representing motion by the combination of a limited number of affine transformations defined locally on a regional division of the space. We show that these transformations not only serve as a first (non-learnt) dimension reduction, but also allow to interpret each of the parameters and relate them to known clinical parameters. Then, we use standard supervised learning algorithms on these parameters to classify the population between infarcted and non-infarcted subjects. The method is applied on the STACOM statistical shape modeling labeled data consisting of 200 cases, comprising the same number of healthy subjects and patients with infarct. We train classifiers using different standard machine learning algorithms. Finally, we validate our method with 10-fold cross-validation and get more than 95 % of correct classification on yet-unseen data. The method is promising and ready to be tested on the remaining 200 test cases of the challenge.

1 Introduction

Myocardial infarction occurs when blood flow to the heart muscle is lowered and the myocardial cells in the territory start dying. The local contractility is reduced and can lead, if prolonged, to severe remodelling of the heart to maintain physiological constraints [1]. The function of the heart is then impaired [2], and is no longer able to pump as efficiently as it used to, which might cause complications. Acute complications may include heart failure if the damaged heart is no longer able to pump blood adequately around the body. Therefore, a quantitative understanding of this pathology and how the heart function changes with an infarct is highly desired. Several methods for computer-aided diagnosis of infarct have already been developed using echocardiographic images of the heart coupled with pattern recognition algorithms [3] although none of the features used are explicitly related to physiological characteristics of cardiac function.

In this article, our goal is to classify between control subjects and patients with infarct in an automatic way, based on the STACOM statistical shape modeling labeled data [4] which consist of a segmentation of the myocardium (both

© Springer International Publishing Switzerland 2016
O. Camara et al. (Eds.): STACOM 2015, LNCS 9534, pp. 190–198, 2016.
DOI: 10.1007/978-3-319-28712-6_21

epi and endo) wall at end-diastole and at end-systole. These two categories of subjects may differ both in the shape of the heart and in the deformation along the cycle. Indeed, after an infarct the damaged region will tend to shrink and the deformation along the cycle will be lower. Similar studies have already been done with the same dataset as [5], which focuses on the shape differences between both population whereas we use both shape and motion features. Due to the complexity and high-dimensionality of these data, we try to quantify both shape and motion using a limited number of parameters, which we combine and use to compare patients and learn the main modes characterizing both populations.

The features of interest characterizing the shape of the patients consist of the regional thickness at both end-diastole and end-systole. We also use features representing the deformation along the cycle. Our approach relies on statistics on the motion of the heart between end-diastole and end-systole. We project the motion on the subspace of polyaffine transformations [6]. With these transformations, we can express a deformation with a limited number of parameters [7]. We develop further the methodology by reducing the transformations to keep only the most relevant parameters.

Then, we test classical machine learning algorithms on our set of combined shape/motion parameters and compare the performance of each algorithm using cross-validation techniques. Validating the method with 10-fold cross-validation, we get results of 95 % correct labeling on yet-unseen cases. In addition, our method notably highlights the relative importance of the different features for the classification of this population.

2   Extraction of Features of Interest Through Shape and Motion Dimensionality Reduction

In this section, we introduce the first dimensionality reduction that is applied to the studied data (made of one segmentation at end-diastole and one at end-systole, each comprised of 1089 points both for the endocardium and the epicardium). It consists in a non-learning approach to project the data of these segmentations to a limited number of regional parameters representing motion and shape.

2.1   Polyaffine Projection

Due to point to point correspondence of the meshes and prior registration, we already have an estimate of the displacement field ϕ mapping each point at end-diastole to the corresponding point at end-systole. Instead of looking at displacements fields, we choose to represent the cardiac motion by the stationary velocity fields (SVF) $\mathbf{v}$ such that $\mathbf{v} = \log \phi$. Working with SVF allows to perform vectorial statistics on diffeomorphisms, while preserving the invertibility constraint, contrary to the Euclidian statistics on displacement fields.

In [6], the authors introduce the space of Log-Euclidean Polyaffine Transformations (LEPT). By defining K regions and smooth weights $\omega_k(x)$, these transformations have the properties to describe locally affine deformations using few parameters while still being invertible. The polyaffine transformation is the weighted sum of these locally-affine transformations $\mathbf{M}_k$:

$$\mathbf{v}_{poly}(x) = \sum_{k=1}^{K} \omega_k(x)\mathbf{M}_k \tilde{x}.$$

In the case of cardiac motion, we have a standardized regional decomposition into the standard American Heart Association (AHA) 17 regions for the left ventricle. We define the weights ω_k as normalized Gaussian functions around the barycenter $\bar{x}_k$ of each region such that:

$$\tilde{\omega}_k(x) = \exp\left(\frac{\kappa}{2}(x - \bar{x}_k)^T \phi_k^{-1}(x - \bar{x}_k)\right), \quad \omega_k(x) = \frac{\tilde{\omega}_k(x)}{\sum_{j=1}^{N} \tilde{\omega}_j(x)}.$$

If we gather the parameters of the polyaffine transformation into a large vector m such that $\mathbf{m} = \text{vect}(\mathbf{M}_1, ..., \mathbf{M}_K)$. The parameters of the optimal projection of a Stationary Velocity Fields $\mathbf{v}$ onto the space of polyaffine transformations has an analytical solution [7] $\mathbf{m} = \hat{\mathbf{m}} = \mathbf{\Sigma}^{-1}b$, which minimizes in the least-squares sense:

$$C(\mathbf{M}_1, ..., \mathbf{M}_K) = \int_\Omega \|v_{poly}(x) - v(x)\|^2 dx \simeq \tfrac{1}{2}(\mathbf{m} - \hat{\mathbf{m}})^T \mathbf{\Sigma}(\mathbf{m} - \hat{\mathbf{m}}) - \tfrac{1}{2}\hat{\mathbf{m}}\mathbf{\Sigma}\hat{\mathbf{m}}.$$

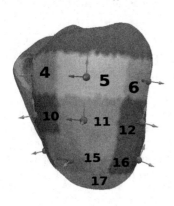

In order to get interpretable parameters for each region, we choose to express them in a local coordinate system adapted to the geometry of the heart. If we call $\mathcal{R} = (\mathbf{O}, \mathbf{e}_1, \mathbf{e}_2, \mathbf{e}_3)$ the original Cartesian coordinate system, we define the local coordinate of the region k as $\mathcal{R}'_i = (\mathbf{O}_k, \mathbf{e}_1^k, \mathbf{e}_2^k, \mathbf{e}_3^k)$ where $\mathbf{O}_k$ is the barycenter of the region (the red point in the enclosed figure), $\mathbf{e}_1$ the radial vector (green vector), $\mathbf{e}_2$ the longitudinal vector (purple vector) and $\mathbf{e}_3$ the circumferential vector (blue vector). We can express the polyaffine parameters $\mathbf{M} = (\mathbf{R}, \mathbf{T})$, where $\mathbf{R}$ is the 3×3 matrix of the rotational parameters and $\mathbf{T}$ is the translation, in this new frame through the equations:

$$\mathbf{R}'_k = \mathbf{P}_k^{-1}\mathbf{R}_k\mathbf{P}_k$$
$$\mathbf{T}'_k = \mathbf{P}_k^{-1}(\mathbf{R}_k\mathbf{O}_k + \mathbf{T}_k),$$

where $\mathbf{P}_k$ is the transfer matrix from the base $(\mathbf{e}_1, \mathbf{e}_2, \mathbf{e}_3)$ to the base $(\mathbf{e}_1^k, \mathbf{e}_2^k, \mathbf{e}_3^k)$. Then, the new expression of the parameters in this local coordinates system:

$$\mathbf{M}_k = \begin{bmatrix} s_r & a_{1,2} & a_{1,3} & t_r \\ a_{2,1} & s_l & a_{2,3} & t_l \\ a_{3,1} & a_{3,2} & s_c & t_c \end{bmatrix},$$

can be related to physiological deformation. The 3 translation parameters correspond to the motion along the 3 local axes (radial, longitudinal, and circumferential) whereas the diagonal coefficients correspond to the strain along these directions.

We propose a method to further reduce the model by keeping only the 3 parameters of the motion and the 3 parameters of the strain. This defines a polyaffine projection that, when expressed in the local basis previously defined, has only these parameters not equal to zero. We first introduce the projection matrix $\mathbf{Q}$ which is a $12K \times 6K$ matrix giving the relation between the $6K$ translation and diagonal parameters expressed in the local coordinates $\mathbf{m_L}$ and the $12K$ parameters expressed in the original coordinates $\mathbf{m}$, such that $\mathbf{Qm_L} = \mathbf{m}$. When expressing $\mathbf{m}$ this way, we constrain it to be within the subspace spanned by $\mathbf{Q}$. This subspace corresponds exactly to the polyaffine transformation whose non-diagonal and non-translation parameters are equal to zero in the local coordinates. The least-square minimization can now be rewritten as:

$$C(\mathbf{m}) \simeq \frac{1}{2}(\mathbf{Qm_L} - \hat{\mathbf{m}})^T \boldsymbol{\Sigma}(\mathbf{Qm_L} - \hat{\mathbf{m}}) - \frac{1}{2}\hat{\mathbf{m}}\boldsymbol{\Sigma}\hat{\mathbf{m}}$$

$$\frac{\partial C}{\partial \mathbf{m_L}} = \mathbf{Q}^T \boldsymbol{\Sigma}(\mathbf{Qm_L} - \hat{\mathbf{m}}) = 0 \implies \mathbf{m} = \mathbf{Qm_L} = \mathbf{Q}(\mathbf{Q}^T\boldsymbol{\Sigma}\mathbf{Q})^{-1}\mathbf{Q}^T\boldsymbol{\Sigma}\hat{\mathbf{m}}$$

For each of the 200 training data we compute the LEPT projection of the deformation field. We are able to parametrize the 3D displacement fields (made of 6534 parameters: 3 parameters for each of the 2178 points of the mesh) by only $6K = 102$ polyaffine parameters. Despite this large reduction of dimensionality, these parameters explain on average more than 70 % of the original displacement. Box-plots of each of the 6 parameters are shown in Fig. 1, where the most discriminant parameters (p value < 0.001) are highlighted in bold. The radial displacement as well as the strain are significantly lower (in absolute value) for the infarcted subjects, which is consistent with what would be clinically expected. Similar differences can be seen for the longitudinal parameters. On the other side, the circumferential motion is less significant, mostly due to the fact that it is very hard to track it accurately with clinical images and therefore not reflected in the provided meshes.

2.2 Thickness Parameters

On top of the polyaffine parameters that characterize the deformation of the heart during a cardiac cycle, we also introduce parameters representing the overall shape of the heart. We choose to study the thickness of the wall within each of the AHA zones at ED and ES. These parameters correspond to the initial and final stages of the transformation from ED to ES, and therefore complement the above-described parameters. We define the thickness as the local distance between endocardial points and their corresponding epicardial locations. These values are also averaged per AHA zone, and summarized in Fig. 2. Significant differences are observed in the thickness of the myocardium wall at end-systole in most of the regions, especially near the apex, for the diseased patients with

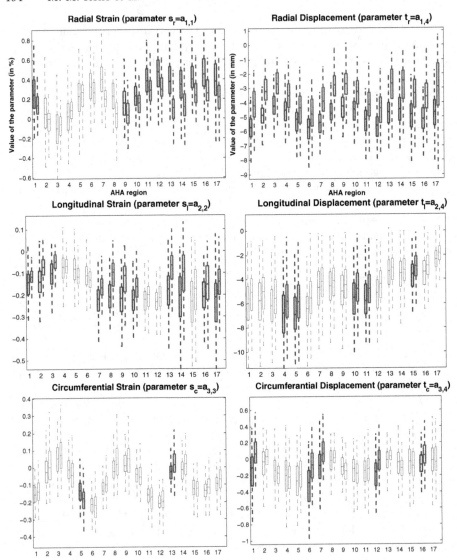

Fig. 1. Parameters of the polyaffine projection both for infarcted patients (red) and control subjects (blue). (Top row): radial parameters for both the diagonal parameters - representing strain - and the translation parameters - representing motion. (Middle row): longitudinal parameters. (Bottom row): circumferential parameters. In bold the most significant parameters (p-value < 0.001) (Color figure online).

respect to the control group. On the other side, thickness ED diastole is less discriminant between both groups. Other parameters related to shape were considered (such as the height of the heart at ED/ES and the diameter at the base at ED/ES) but no significant differences between both populations were seen and therefore we do not use them for classification.

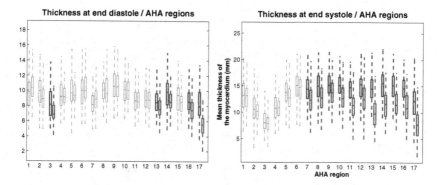

Fig. 2. Box-plots of the thickness of the myocardium wall per AHA region. In blue, the control set and in red the patients with infarcts. (Left): end-diastole. (Right): end-systole. In bold the most significant parameters (p-value < 0.001) (Color figure online).

3 Dimensionality Reduction of the Parameters and Classification

In this section, we use both polyaffine and thickness parameters previously introduced in order to classify between healthy and infarcted subjects. We use the machine-learning toolbox Scikit-Learn [8] to test a collection of standard state-of-the-art algorithms on our dataset and compare their performance in predicting yet unseen data. The features that serve to feed the tested learned algorithms were considered in four different ways: either polyaffine or thickness parameters separately (sets # 1 and # 2), or concatenated without normalization (# 3) or with normalization so that they have a mean of 0 and a variance of 1.

3.1 Learnt Dimensionality Reduction

Complementary to the a-priori reduction of dimensionality imposed by the polyaffine model and the use of 17 AHA regions, we also evaluated the influence of a second dimensionality reduction of the data both with a Principal Component Analysis (PCA) and a Principal Least Square (PLS) decomposition [9] prior to the tested algorithm. PCA is designed to spread the data according to the main modes of variability and is known to be a useful dimension reduction pre-processing to prevent over-fitting and improve the performance of some machine-learning algorithm. PLS looks at modes of the input variables that correlate the most with an output variable (in our case the pathology label 0 or 1). Therefore, in contrast with PCA, the modes also correlate with our classification. In particular, Fig. 3 summarizes the loadings of the first mode of the PLS with respect to each parameter. Notably, this can be used to assess which of the parameters is the most important for the classification. The radial parameters are the most prevalent, whereas both the circumferential parameters and the thickness at ED provide very little contribution to the first mode and therefore the classification.

			STRAIN			TRANSLATION			THICKNESS		SUM OVER ALL PARAMETERS
									END DIASTOLE	END SYSTOLE	
			RADIAL	LONG	CIRC	RADIAL	LONG	CIRC			
AHA REGIONS	BASE	1	0.9%	0.3%	0.0%	2.1%	0.9%	0.5%	0.0%	0.2%	5%
		2	0.4%	0.9%	0.0%	2.3%	0.9%	0.1%	0.2%	0.2%	5%
		3	0.0%	0.6%	0.0%	2.0%	1.2%	0.0%	0.3%	0.2%	4%
		4	0.0%	0.0%	0.2%	1.5%	1.3%	0.0%	0.0%	0.0%	3%
		5	0.1%	0.1%	0.3%	1.2%	1.2%	0.2%	0.0%	0.2%	3%
		6	0.5%	0.0%	0.0%	1.5%	1.0%	0.5%	0.0%	0.2%	4%
	MIDDLE	7	1.9%	1.4%	0.2%	2.3%	0.8%	0.5%	0.0%	0.8%	8%
		8	1.3%	1.6%	0.2%	2.6%	0.9%	0.0%	0.0%	0.8%	7%
		9	0.9%	1.6%	0.1%	2.4%	1.1%	0.1%	0.0%	0.6%	7%
		10	0.8%	1.3%	0.0%	1.9%	1.2%	0.0%	0.0%	0.7%	6%
		11	0.9%	0.5%	0.0%	1.5%	1.2%	0.0%	0.0%	0.7%	5%
		12	1.5%	0.6%	0.0%	1.7%	1.0%	0.4%	0.0%	0.6%	6%
	APICAL	13	1.9%	1.3%	0.4%	2.5%	0.8%	0.1%	0.3%	1.6%	9%
		14	1.6%	1.2%	0.2%	2.2%	1.0%	0.1%	0.2%	1.2%	8%
		15	1.4%	0.7%	0.0%	1.6%	1.1%	0.0%	0.1%	1.1%	6%
		16	1.7%	0.7%	0.1%	1.8%	0.9%	0.4%	0.3%	1.1%	7%
	APEX	17	1.2%	1.1%	0.4%	1.5%	1.0%	0.0%	0.6%	1.1%	7%
SUM OVER ALL REGIONS			17.0%	13.8%	2.2%	32.7%	17.8%	3.0%	2.1%	11.4%	

Fig. 3. Loadings of the first PLS mode showing the contribution of each of the parameters and each of the AHA zone. In green the most important parameters and in red the less important (Color figure online).

3.2 Classification

All algorithms were tested with 10-fold cross validation on the dataset made of 200 patients. Figure 4 summarizes the results of the different algorithms. Combining both sets of parameters improves the performance of most of the algorithms showing that these sets give different kind of information about the data. We also see that PLS regression, by preprocessing the data and orienting

		Decision Tree	Random Forest	Logistic Regression	Nearest Neighbors	SVM Linear	SVM svc
	PolyAffine (PA)	79%	88%	85%	81%	89%	86%
	Thickness (TH)	76%	84%	86%	89%	85%	86%
	PA + TH	79%	91%	89%	90%	90%	92%
	Norm. PA + TH	77%	88%	92%	85%	90%	94%
PCA	2 Modes	84%	87%	90%	89%	87%	89%
	5 Modes	84%	87%	90%	87%	88%	93%
	10 Modes	84%	89%	90%	87%	88%	93%
	All modes	84%	80%	93%	87%	92%	96%
PLS	2 Modes	91%	93%	94%	94%	93%	94%
	5 Modes	91%	96%	96%	97%	95%	97%
	10 Modes	91%	97%	96%	94%	95%	96%
	All modes	91%	94%	94%	94%	93%	94%

Fig. 4. Cross-validation results (10-fold) of the classification with respect to different state-of-the-art machine learning algorithms and different sets of input data. Combination of algorithms and parameters that have the best performance are shown in green whereas the worst are shown in red (Color figure online).

the modes of the input variables upto the best correlation with the pathology labels, improves the performance of all machine learning algorithms especially for Decision Tree and Nearest Neighbors. With more than 95 % of correct labeling, SVM-SVC algorithm used on the PLS reduction with 5 modes is the method that performs the best. It is interesting to see that increasing the number of PLS modes further does not improve the classification. Our interpretation is that the subsequent modes of the PLS are not correlated to the classification and can therefore induce over-fitting of the data. We also tested the method with different cross-validation such as leave-one-out, 2-fold or 5-fold in order to see the robustness of the method with respect to the size of the training set and got similar performance.

4 Conclusion

In this paper, we evaluated the contribution of prior reduction of dimensionality to the classification of high-dimensional motion data. One of the assets of our work is an innovative methodology to project a motion on a reduced number of polyaffine parameters. We apply the methodology to classify a population and detect an infarct based on the segmentations at end-systole and end-diastole. Following the first dimensionality reduction given by the polyaffine parameters, we use traditional statistical reductions on our sets of parameters with PCA and PLS. Using 10-fold cross validation, we show that the resulting parameters have good predictive power with more than 95 % correct classification on 200 infarcted/control cases. We are also able to quantify the importance of each of the parameters in the classification. Notably, this provides insights into what is the main impact of an infarct both in terms of motion and shape.

Ackowledgements. The authors acknowledge the partial funding by the EU FP7-funded project MD-Paedigree (Grant Agreement 600932).

References

1. Konstam, M.A., Kramer, D.G., Patel, A.R., Maron, M.S., Udelson, J.E.: Left ventricular remodeling in heart failure: current concepts in clinical significance and assessment. JACC: Cardiovasc. Imaging **4**, 98–108 (2011)
2. Bijnens, B., Claus, P., Weidemann, F., Strotmann, J., Sutherland, G.: Investigating cardiac function using motion and deformation analysis in the setting of coronary artery disease. Circulation **116**, 2453–2464 (2007)
3. Sudarshan, V., Acharya, U.R., Yin-Kwee Ng, E., Meng, C.S., Tan, R.S., Ghista, D.N.: Automated identification of infarcted myocardium tissue characterisation using ultrasound images: a review. IEEE Rev. Biomed. Eng. **8**, 86–97 (2013)
4. Fonseca, C., Backhaus, M., Bluemke, D., Britten, R., Chung, J., Cowan, B., Dinov, I., Finn, J., Hunter, P., Kadish, A., Lee, D., Lima, J., Medrano-Gracia, P., Shivkumar, K., Suinesiaputra, A., Tao, W., Young, A.: The cardiac atlas project-an imaging database for computational modeling and statistical atlases of the heart. Bioinformatics **27**(5), 2288–2295 (2011). 2011-08-15 00:00:00.0

5. Zhang, X., et al.: Orthogonal shape modes describing clinical indices of remodeling. In: van Assen, H., Bovendeerd, P., Delhaas, T. (eds.) FIMH 2015. LNCS, vol. 9126, pp. 273–281. Springer, Heidelberg (2015)
6. Arsigny, V., Commowick, O., Ayache, N., Pennec, X.: A fast and log-euclidean polyaffine framework for locally linear registration. J. Math. Imaging Vis. **33**, 222–238 (2009)
7. McLeod, K., Sermesant, M., Beerbaum, P., Pennec, X.: Spatio-temporal tensor decomposition of a polyaffine motion model for a better analysis of pathological left ventricular dynamics. IEEE Trans. Med. Imaging **34**, 1562–1575 (2015)
8. Pedregosa, F., Varoquaux, G., Gramfort, A., Michel, V., Thirion, B., Grisel, O., Blondel, M., Prettenhofer, P., Weiss, R., Dubourg, V., Vanderplas, J., Passos, A., Cournapeau, D., Brucher, M., Perrot, M., Duchesnay, E.: Scikit-learn: Machine learning in Python. J. Mach. Learn. Res. **12**, 2825–2830 (2011)
9. Rosipal, R., Krämer, N.C.: Overview and recent advances in partial least squares. In: Saunders, C., Grobelnik, M., Gunn, S., Shawe-Taylor, J. (eds.) SLSFS 2005. LNCS, vol. 3940, pp. 34–51. Springer, Heidelberg (2006)

Automatic Detection of Cardiac Remodeling Using Global and Local Clinical Measures and Random Forest Classification

Jan Ehrhardt[1]([⊠]), Matthias Wilms[1], Heinz Handels[1], and Dennis Säring[2,3]

[1] Institute of Medical Informatics, University of Lübeck, Lübeck, Germany
{ehrhardt,wilms,handels}@imi.uni-luebeck.de
[2] Department of Computational Neuroscience,
University Medical Center Hamburg-Eppendorf, Hamburg, Germany
dsg@fh-wedel.de
[3] University of Applied Sciences, Wedel, Germany

Abstract. Myocardial infarction leads to a change in geometry and a modified motion characteristics of the heart, called remodeling. The detection of patients with subclinical remodeling is clinically relevant because effective therapies have to be initiated early to avoid a progressive dilatation, and deterioration in contractile function.

In this paper, we propose a classification approach to detect patients with cardiac remodeling based on established global and local clinical parameters, like end-diastolic and end-systolic volume, ejection fraction or local myocardial thickness. The functional parameters are extracted based on segmented endo- and epicardial contours using an in-house developed software tool. A random decision forest is trained for recognition of patients with impaired shape or motion characteristics. The 17 segment model of the left ventricle proposed by the American Heart Association is compared to a higher resolution model using 97 left ventricle segments in terms of classification performance.

The classification results are submitted to the left ventricle statistical shape modelling challenge with the aim to compare the classification performance of classical clinical parameters with other probabilistic or model-based approaches. A leave-one-out cross-validation shows an accuracy of 0.93 using global and local parameters compared to an accuracy of 0.86 using global parameters only.

Keywords: Computer aided diagnosis · Cardiac remodeling · Myocardial infarction · Random decision forests

1 Introduction

Myocardial infarction is the leading cause of death for both men and women in the western civilization. The quality of life and the course of disease for patients

---

www.cardiacatlas.org/web/stacom2015/statistical-shape-challenge.

© Springer International Publishing Switzerland 2016
O. Camara et al. (Eds.): STACOM 2015, LNCS 9534, pp. 199–207, 2016.
DOI: 10.1007/978-3-319-28712-6_22

depends on the revitalization of the myocardium and avoiding the development of a persistent dysfunctional contraction of the heart, which can lead to progressive impairment of the heart function combined with cardiac remodeling. Early detection of patients with risk of remodeling is clinically relevant to initiate effective therapies early to avoid remodeling.

The *left ventricle (LV) statistical shape modelling challenge: myocardial infarction* aims to compare probabilistic models for myocardial impairment detection. Based on a training set of LV shapes, participants are called to generate classification models to distinguish between normal and abnormal cases. Diagnosis of myocardial infarction is usually based on multiple MRI sequences (e.g. cine-MRI and LGE-MRI). Several clinical parameters, like LV mass and volume, ejection fraction (EF) or relative infarct size, are used to grade the impairment. Beside those global functional parameters, the 17 segment model recommended by the American Heart Association (AHA) is widely used for the visual interpretation of regional LV abnormalities [4]. Local functional parameters, like LV wall motion and thickness, can be visually assessed on a 17-segments bull's-eye display.

Several approaches exist for automatic detection of LV motion abnormalities based on LV segmentations, including methods based on statistical shape models (SSMs) [2,17,21], Bayesian or neural networks [14,18,20], information theoretic measures [13] or classification methods [5]. Studies show a disagreement of up to 30 % between SSM-based methods and visual LV wall motion scores (VWMS) [17]. Besides inaccuracies in the model approaches, this is due to the subjectivity and large inter-observer variability of VWMS [12] and because segment-based scoring may underestimate motion abnormalities near segment borders.

The aim of our approach is to detect patients with cardiac remodeling based on established clinical functional parameters. Previous studies compared the classification performance of SSM-based or information theoretic methods against traditional clinical indicators of remodeling [13,17,21], however, in these studies only global clinical parameters were analyzed. In contrast, in our approach global and local clinical parameters are computed based on provided end-diastolic (ED) and end-systolic (ES) shapes of the endo- and epicardium. The computed measures are used to train a classifier for the detection of LV motion abnormalities/cardiac remodeling. We hypothesize that local functional parameters improve the performance of LV motion abnormality detection. The aim of our contribution within the scope of this challenge is to compare directly the classification performance of these parameters with other probabilistic or model-based approaches.

In our study, two hundred ED and ES shapes provided by the challenge are used to extract functional parameters. The extracted parameters are used for the supervised training of random forests [3] with extremely randomized trees [7] for the recognition of LV motion abnormalities. To investigate the influence of the parameters, experiments are performed using global parameters, local parameters based on the 17 segment model, and local parameters with higher spatial resolution as suggested in [15,16].

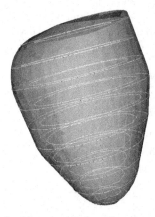

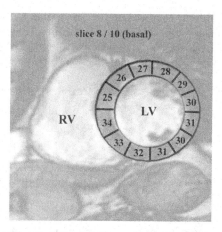

Fig. 1. 10 epicardial and endocardial contours extracted from a triangulated shape of the left ventricle.

Fig. 2. Visualization of the segment model with higher spatial resolution for one basal slice. Segments 25 and 26 belong to segment 2 of the AHA model, segments 27 and 28 belong to AHA segment 1 and so on.

A leave-one-out cross-validation is performed on the training data to estimate the classification performance.

2   Methods

The aim of our approach is to compare the classification performance of methods provided by other challenge-participants against the performance of classical clinical parameters. Therefore, we aspire to imitate the clinical workflow with the provided challenge data and our *Heart Analysis Tool* (HeAT) [11,15] to compute the clinical measures. In the following sections, the necessary preprocessing of the challenge data and the computation of parameters is explained in detail.

2.1   Preprocessing of the Shape Data

In clinical praxis, the diagnosis of LV shape and motion is frequently based on endocardial and epicardial contours extracted from cine-MRI sequences. To imitate image-based input data from the given training shapes, the triangulated surface models are converted to contours by placing 10 cut planes between the most basal and most apical points on the ED surface, leading to realistic slice distances of 8–13 mm (mean: 10 mm, see Fig. 1). The resulting contour points are interpolated with 2D Beziér-Spline functions to generate smooth continuous contours per slice.

Table 1. Comparison between global LV function parameters for one hundred asymptomatic cases (MESA) and one hundred patients with myocardial infarction (DETERMINE). (EDV: end-diastolic volume; ESV: end- systolic volume; SV: stroke volume; LVEF: left ventricular ejection fraction; Mass: mass of the myocardium).

Measure	MESA	DETERMINE
EDV [ml]	104 ± 28	165 ± 45
ESV [ml]	40 ± 18	92 ± 38
SV [ml]	64 ± 20	72 ± 29
LVEF [%]	61 ± 13	45 ± 15
Mass [g]	123 ± 47	155 ± 48

2.2   Computation of Global and Local Parameters

The generated contours are imported into our in-house software system for the analysis of cardiac MRI sequences to compute clinical parameters [15]. Time and intensity related measures as well as infarct size can not be computed, because image data are not provided and ED+ES phase of endocard and epicard are given only. Table 1 compares the five computed global functional parameters of asymptomatic cases and of patients with myocardial infarction given in the training set.

The software system offers two modes of local parameter computation: the 17 segment model and a model with a higher number of segments based on the centerline method [16]. For both models, corresponding points in the middle of the septum (provided with the challenge data) are used to define corresponding segments across all patients. To define the model with higher spatial resolution, a centerline is computed based on the epicardial contours and each segment of the 17 segment model is subdivided into 6 evenly spaced segments, except the apex (see Fig. 2). Thus, 97 segments are defined while the anatomical mapping based on the coronary artery blood supply is preserved.

For each segment the following four local parameters are computed: myocardial wall thickness as the absolute difference between endocardial and epicardial contour position in ED, change in wall thickness between ES and ED, and motion amplitude of the endocardium as the magnitude of the movement between ES and ED of the endocardial contour. The last local parameter describes the symmetric or asymmetric contraction of the endocardium ES to ED regarding to the center of mass of the LV. In total 68 local parameters are computed for each training case using the 17 segment model and 388 for the model with higher resolution (the apex is excluded in both models).

2.3   Supervised Classification Using Random Forests

We choose to use random decision forests (RDFs) [3,8] to classify into asymptomatic cases and infarct patients based on the computed global and local parameters. RDFs are an ensemble of decision trees, where each decision tree is trained on a subset of the training samples and a subset of the available features (here: functional parameters) using a splitting strategy at each node. Based on the decisions of the individual trees, the RDF predicts the class probabilities of a test sample. In our two-class problem a threshold t is needed to assign each test sample to one of the classes "asymptomatic" or "infarct".

RDFs are known to be accurate, robust, fast, scalable and easy to use. Compared to logistic regression, RDFs do not expect the features to be roughly linear or the problem to be linearly separable. Further, RDFs provide methods to evaluate the importance of features. However, in our application many features are highly correlated (e.g. EDV and ESV) and classical methods for feature ranking may be misleading [19].

The main parameters of RDFs are the number of trees N in the forests, the maximum depth d_{max} of each tree and the splitting strategy. Extremely randomized trees (Extra-Trees) [7] are used as splitting strategy in our application. Extra-Trees had shown to have a higher computational efficiency and accuracy for different types of classification problems [7].

2.4 Experiments and Evaluation

Three experiments are performed in our study. In the first experiment only global functional parameters are used to train the RDF classifier. The second experiment additionally uses local parameters based on the 17 segment model, and in the third experiment, we extract the local parameters with higher spatial resolution to investigate the influence of the segment-based averaging.

Two hundred ED and ES shapes provided by the challenge are used for a leave-one-out cross-validation to estimate the classification performance. The goodness of fit for each of the three experiments is compared qualitatively using receiver operating characteristic, and quantitatively by the area under the curve and accuracy of the trained classifiers.

3 Results

The provided training dataset comprises one hundred cases with myocardial infarction and an additional one hundred asymptomatic cases from the DETERMINE and MESA datasets respectively [1,9], contributed to the Cardiac Atlas Project [6]. For each case, triangulated shapes at end-diastole (ED) and end-systole (ES) are provided with point-wise inter- and intra-subject correspondence.

All cases in the training data set are processed as described in Sect. 2.1 and global and local functional parameters are extracted. The average global functional parameters are summarized in Table 1. A heteroscedastic two-sided t-test reveals significant differences between the groups for all global parameters except SV ($p < 0.005$). Comparison with EDV, ESV and Mass provided in [21] suggests that the global parameters are slightly underestimated, possibly due to the conversion into slice-wise contours.

Table 2. Results of the leave-one-out cross-validation using 200 training shapes: area-under-the-curve (AUC), accuracy, specificity and sensitivity for the three experiments.

	AUC	accuracy $(t=0.5)$	specificity $(t=0.5)$	sensitivity $(t=0.5)$
Experiment 1 (global parameters)	0.92	0.86	0.87	0.86
Experiment 2 (global + local parameters, 17 segment model)	0.96	0.90	0.90	0.90
Experiment 3 (global + local parameters, 97 segment model)	0.97	0.93	0.93	0.92

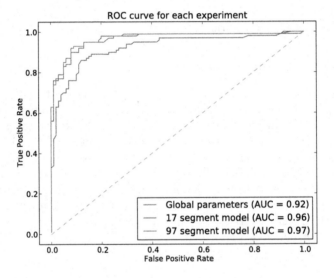

Fig. 3. Receiver operating characteristic (ROC) for each of the three experiments.

A RDF with $N = 400$ decision trees and $d_{max} = 50$ was trained using the global functional parameters (experiment 1), global and local parameters extracted by the 17 segment model (experiment 2), and global and local parameters extracted by the higher resolution model (experiment 3). The RDF parameters were optimized using grid search and cross-validation. However, we found the classification performance to be relatively insensitive to parameter variations.

Leave-one-out cross-validation was performed on the training data to estimate the performance of our classification approach. By varying the threshold t, specificity and sensitivity of the classifier can be adjusted. Receiver operating characteristic (ROC) comparing the three experiments are shown in Fig. 3. The natural choice of $t = 0.5$ leads to a classification accuracy of 0.93 for the 97 segment model. Table 2 compares area under the ROC curve (AUC), accuracy,

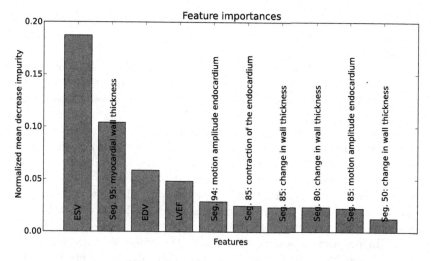

Fig. 4. The 10 most important features in terms of normalized mean decrease impurity [10] of a 97 segment model-RDF trained on all 200 training cases.

sensitivity, and specificity for each of the three experiments. The results show that experiment 2 and 3 achieved a better performance than experiment 1. The 97 segment model performed slightly better than the 17 segment model.

Figure 4 exemplary shows the 10 most important features in terms of mean decrease impurity of a RDF trained by using the 97 segment model and all 200 training cases. It is interesting to note that 3 of the top 4 parameters are global markers (ESV, EDV, and LVEF) and that segment 85 appears three times in the top ten. Segment 85 is laterally located in the apical region (second slice) and is part of segment 16 in the 17 segment model. In general, it has to be noted that many features are highly correlated (e.g. EDV and ESV), which limits the interpretability of the ranking.

The challenge provides an additional test data set comprising two hundred cases with unknown ground truth. The global and local parameters computed with the 97 segment model were used to obtain the results for the test data that were finally submitted as challenge entry (HeAT-RDF).

4   Discussion and Conclusions

We have proposed a classification scheme based on global and local functional cardiac parameters to distinguish between asymptomatic LV motion and patients with myocardial infarction. Due to the unavailability of image data, only end-diastolic and end-systolic shapes of the left ventricle were used to extract classical global and regional clinical parameters for LV motion diagnosis. To address the limited spatial resolution of the AHA 17 segment model, regional functional parameters were extracted using a 97 segment model, too. Both models were compared to a model solely based on global parameters in terms of classification performance. The extracted global and regional parameters were used to train a random decision forest with Extra-Trees based an two hundred training samples. A leave-one-out cross-validation was performed to evaluate the performance of our classification approach.

The accuracy of 0.93 and AUC of 0.97 of the proposed classification approach is comparable with values reported for other MRI-based infarct classification methods, including SSM-based methods [17,21] or a method based on information theoretic measures [13]. However, comparability of the reported values is limited due to the differences in image data, sample sizes and ground truth reliability. Few methods were published that clearly outperform the proposed method. An AUC of 0.99 was reported in [21], however, additional meta data, like age, sex and weight were available in this study.

Further, we have shown that the inclusion of local functional parameters increases the classification performance and a higher resolution of local functional parameters performs slightly better compared to the 17 segment model.

The main purpose of our contribution in the scope of this challenge is to compare the classification ability of classical clinical parameters with shape-model based methods provided by other challenge participants, and thus to help to assess the reliability of these clinical measures.

Acknowledgments. This work was supported by the German Research Foundation (DFG, EH 224/6-1).

References

1. Bild, D.E., Bluemke, D.A., Burke, G.L., Detrano, R., Roux, A.V.D., Folsom, A.R., Greenland, P., Jacobs Jr., D.R., Kronmal, R., Liu, K., et al.: Multi-ethnic study of atherosclerosis: objectives and design. Am. J. Epidemiol. **156**(9), 871–881 (2002)
2. Bosch, J.G., Nijland, F., Mitchell, S.C., Lelieveldt, B.P., Kamp, O., Reiber, J.H., Sonka, M.: Computer-aided diagnosis via model-based shape analysis: automated classification of wall motion abnormalities in echocardiograms. Acad. Radiol. **12**(3), 358–367 (2005)
3. Breiman, L.: Random forests. Mach. Learn. **45**(1), 5–32 (2001)
4. Cerqueira, M.D., Weissman, N.J., Dilsizian, V., Jacobs, A.K., Kaul, S., Laskey, W.K., Pennell, D.J., Rumberger, J.A., Ryan, T., Verani, M.S.: Standardized myocardial segmentation and nomenclature for tomographic imaging of the heart: a statement for healthcare professionals from the cardiac imaging committee of the council on clinical cardiology of the american heart association. Circulation **105**(4), 539–542 (2002)
5. Chykeyuk, K., Clifton, D., Noble, J.A., et al.: Feature extraction and wall motion classification of 2d stress echocardiography with relevance vector machines. In: 2011 IEEE International Symposium on Biomedical Imaging: From Nano to Macro, pp. 677–680. IEEE (2011)
6. Fonseca, C.G., Backhaus, M., Bluemke, D.A., Britten, R.D., Chung, J.D., Cowan, B.R., Dinov, I.D., Finn, J.P., Hunter, P.J., Kadish, A.H., Lee, D.C., Lima, J.A.C., Medrano-Gracia, P., Shivkumar, K., Suinesiaputra, A., Tao, W., Young, A.A.: The cardiac atlas project - an imaging database for computational modeling and statistical atlases of the heart. Bioinformatics **27**(16), 2288–2295 (2011)

7. Geurts, P., Ernst, D., Wehenkel, L.: Extremely randomized trees. Mach. Learn. **63**(1), 3–42 (2006)
8. Ho, T.K.: The random subspace method for constructing decision forests. IEEE Trans. Pattern Anal. Mach. Intell. **20**(8), 832–844 (1998)
9. Kadish, A.H., Bello, D., Finn, J., Bonow, R.O., Schaechter, A., Subacius, H., Albert, C., Daubert, J.P., Fonseca, C.G., Goldberger, J.J.: Rationale and design for the defibrillators to reduce risk by magnetic resonance imaging evaluation (determine) trial. J. Cardiovasc. Electrophysiol. **20**(9), 982–987 (2009)
10. Louppe, G., Wehenkel, L., Sutera, A., Geurts, P.: Understanding variable importances in forests of randomized trees. In: Advances in Neural Information Processing Systems, pp. 431–439 (2013)
11. Lund, G., Saering, D., Muellerleile, K., Cuerlis, J., Barz, D., Bannas, P., Radunski, U.K., Sydow, K., Adam, G.: Evaluation of a new semi-automatic strategy for quantitative measurement of infarct size in patients with acute and chronic myocardial infarction using cardiac magnetic resonance imaging. J. Cardiovasc. Magn. Reson. **15**(1), P201 (2013)
12. Paetsch, I., Jahnke, C., Ferrari, V.A., Rademakers, F.E., Pellikka, P.A., Hundley, W.G., Poldermans, D., Bax, J.J., Wegscheider, K., Fleck, E., et al.: Determination of interobserver variability for identifying inducible left ventricular wall motion abnormalities during dobutamine stress magnetic resonance imaging. Eur. Heart J. **27**(12), 1459–1464 (2006)
13. Punithakumar, K., Ben Ayed, I., Ross, I.G., Islam, A., Chong, J., Li, S.: Detection of left ventricular motion abnormality via information measures and bayesian filtering. IEEE Trans. Inf. Technol. Biomed. **14**(4), 1106–1113 (2010)
14. Qazi, M., Fung, G., Krishnan, S., Rosales, R., Steck, H., Rao, R.B., Poldermans, D., Chandrasekaran, D.: Automated heart wall motion abnormality detection from ultrasound images using bayesian networks. IJCAI **7**, 519–525 (2007)
15. Säring, D., Ehrhardt, J., Stork, A., Bansmann, M., Lund, G., Handels, H.: Computer-assisted analysis of 4D cardiac MR image sequences after myocardial infarction. Methods Inf. Med. **45**(4), 377–383 (2006)
16. Sheehan, F.H., Bolson, E.L., Dodge, H.T., Mathey, D.G., Schofer, J., Woo, H.: Advantages and applications of the centerline method for characterizing regional ventricular function. Circulation **74**(2), 293–305 (1986)
17. Suinesiaputra, A., Frangi, A., Kaandorp, T., Lamb, H., Bax, J., Reiber, J., Lelieveldt, B.: Automated detection of regional wall motion abnormalities based on a statistical model applied to multislice short-axis cardiac mr images. IEEE Trans. Med. Imaging **28**(4), 595–607 (2009)
18. Then, J., Raman, V., Patrick Then, H.H., Enn Ong, S.E.: Literature review and proposed framework on CAD: automated cardiac MR images segmentation and classification. In: Papasratorn, B., Charoenkitkarn, N., Lavangnananda, K., Chutimaskul, W., Vanijja, V. (eds.) IAIT 2012. CCIS, vol. 344, pp. 170–180. Springer, Heidelberg (2012)
19. Tolosi, L., Lengauer, T.: Classification with correlated features: unreliability of feature ranking and solutions. Bioinformatics **27**(14), 1986–1994 (2011)
20. Tsai, D.Y., Sekiya, M., Lee, Y.: Computer-aided diagnosis in abdominal and cardiac radiology using neural networks. In: Proceedings of the IEEE International Conference on Neural Information Processing. Citeseer (2001)
21. Zhang, X., Cowan, B.R., Bluemke, D.A., Finn, J.P., Fonseca, C.G., Kadish, A.H., Lee, D.C., Lima, J.A., Suinesiaputra, A., Young, A.A., et al.: Atlas-based quantification of cardiac remodeling due to myocardial infarction. PLoS One **9**(10), e110243 (2014)

Automatic Detection of Myocardial Infarction Through a Global Shape Feature Based on Local Statistical Modeling

Mahdi Tabassian[1,2]([envelope]) , Martino Alessandrini[2], Peter Claes[3],
Luca De Marchi[1], Dirk Vandermeulen[3], Guido Masetti[1], and Jan D'hooge[2]

[1] Department of Electrical, Electronic and Information Engineering,
University of Bologna, Bologna, Italy
`mahdi.tabassian2@unibo.it`
[2] Department of Cardiovascular Sciences,
Laboratory on Cardiovascular Imaging and Dynamics,
KU Leuven, Leuven, Belgium
[3] Department of Electrical Engineering–ESAT,
Medical Imaging Research Center (MIRC), KU Leuven, Leuven, Belgium

Abstract. This paper presents a local-to-global statistical approach for modeling the major components of left ventricular (LV) shape using its 3-D landmark representation. The rationale for dividing the LV into local areas is bi-fold: (1) to better identify abnormalities that lead to local shape remodeling and, (2) to decrease the number of shape variables by using a limited set of landmark points for an efficient statistical parametrization. Principal Component Analysis (PCA) is used for the statistical modeling of the local regions and subsets of the learned parameters that provide significant discriminatory information are taken from each local model in a feature selection stage. The selected local parameters are then concatenated to form a global representation of the LV and to train a classifier for differentiating between normal and infarcted LV shapes.

Keywords: Local statistical shape modeling · Principal component analysis · Feature selection · Myocardial abnormality detection

1 Introduction

Statistical shape analysis is a promising approach to model cardiac anatomy and to characterize myocardial abnormalities. The success of the point distribution model (PDM) [2] in describing anatomical structures of medical images makes it the basis of the majority of cardiac shape parametrization algorithms. These algorithms have been established using both linear methods (such as Principal Component Analysis (PCA) [7,12,14,18] and Independent Component Analysis (ICA) [15]) and nonlinear techniques (such as kernel PCA [5]). One drawback of these techniques, however, is that they treat the shape globally. In addition to being computationally expensive due to the requirement of modeling a large

© Springer International Publishing Switzerland 2016
O. Camara et al. (Eds.): STACOM 2015, LNCS 9534, pp. 208–216, 2016.
DOI: 10.1007/978-3-319-28712-6_23

number of variables, a global approach may fail to characterize abnormalities that affect small regions of the myocardium. An alternative approach is to learn local statistical shape components and then merge their results to describe the global shape as a poly-local model. A recent and well-established example of such framework is presented in [17]. It is based on utilizing local shape descriptors, but not landmark points as suggested in PDM, and employing a manifold learning technique called ISOMAP [16] for dimension reduction.

Inspired by [17], a local statistical shape modeling approach based on PDM and PCA [9] is presented in this paper to characterize major components of LV shapes. The rationale of utilizing PCA in our framework is as follows: (1) PCA implementation involves simple steps and its parameters can be efficiently computed and, (2) it allows to visualize major modes of data variation. The latter property could be of particular interest to study the relation between the parameters of the statistical model and the patho-physiology of the heart.

The main contribution of this paper compared to the framework presented in [17] is the way that the local statistical information are incorporated in the classification phase. In [17], an independent classifier was built with the parameters of each local model and the classifiers' decisions were fused using majority voting. Independent treatment of the local models' parameters could degrade the capability of the combined classification model in dealing with abnormalities that affect small regions of the heart. Here, we propose to create an alternative local-to-global representation of the LV shape components by concatenating the parameters of the local models and then building a classifier with the obtained feature vector. Having the advantage of encoding global shape parameters of the LV, the spatial relation between the local zones is taken into consideration using this technique. Explicit usage of the local statistical parameters can also create distinct areas in the global feature space. This property enables a classification system to better characterize abnormalities that mostly affect small regions of the myocardium.

2   Materials and Methods

Figure 1 represents global and local architectures that were implemented in this paper for the statistical modeling and classification of LV shapes. In the local architecture (Fig. 1(b)), the LV was divided into non-overlapping regions of interest (ROI) and an independent PCA model was built with the local shapes belonging to each ROI. By taking a subset of the learned statistical parameters, two different classification schemes were examined. In addition, a global PCA model (Fig. 1(a)) was also built to benchmark the performances of the local PCA models.

2.1   Data and Preprocessing

A data set of 100 healthy volunteers and 100 patients with myocardial infarction from the MESA [1] and DETERMINE studies [10] respectively, was used in

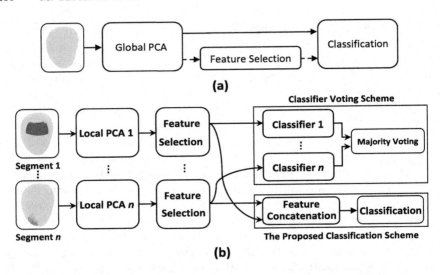

Fig. 1. Architectures of the implemented statistical frameworks. (a) A PCA model is constructed with whole LV shapes. Then, a subset of the first PCs (solid line) or selected PCs (dashed line) is used for training a classifier. (b) Independent PCA models are built with the segments of LV shapes and subsets of the selected PCs are used in the classification phase. In the classifier voting scheme, independent classifiers are trained with the selected PCs of the local models and the final decision is made by the majority voting rule. In the proposed scheme, one classifier is trained with a feature vector that is obtained by concatenating the local models' parameters.

our experiments. These data sets are part of the Cardiac Atlas Project (CAP, www.cardiacatlas.org) [6] and contain cardiovascular magnetic resonance (CMR) images. Endocardial and epicardial shapes at end-diastole (ED) and end-systole (ES) are represented with their corresponding Cartesian sets of landmark points in magnet coordinates. It has been demonstrated in [18] that a PCA model built with shape vectors at ED and ES could provide better outcomes than its counterparts that were constructed with only ED or ES shapes. Therefore, the shapes of both ED and ES cardiac phases were used for the implementation of the global and local PCA models in the current study.

All shapes were aligned by making use of the generalized Procrustes superimposition method [13]. As suggested in [18], for building the global PCA model the alignment phase has been performed by eliminating position and orientation differences but preserving scale variations as ventricular size has a predictive value for diagnosing myocardial infarction. For constructing the local PCA models, however, scale variations were also removed in the alignment procedure.

2.2   Statistical Modeling

Both global and local PCA models were learned using the data of the healthy volunteers to capture major modes of normal shape variations. For building the local PCA models, small, medium and large ROI sizes were examined which respectively encompassed 4, 8 and 16 faces of the 3-D meshes in both the circumferential and longitudinal directions where the full LV mesh was composed of 32×32 faces. Note that the landmark points in each ROI were consistent across the subjects.

2.3 Feature Selection

The ultimate goal of the presented framework is the accurate categorization of the normal and infarcted LV shapes. This requires that the statistical parameters taken for training a classification system provide significant discriminatory information. Traditionally, data are projected onto the subspace spanned by the first principal components (PCs) to retain most of the variation in the original variables. However, it is possible that some of the PCs with low contribution in the data variation contain relevant discriminatory information. As such, the P-metric method [8] was used in our framework to select relevant PCs:

$$P(PC_i) = \frac{|\mu_{i1} - \mu_{i2}|}{\sigma_{i1} + \sigma_{i2}} \qquad (1)$$

where μ_{i1} and μ_{i2} are respectively the means of the normal and infarcted samples after projecting onto the subspace of the ith PC and σ_{i1} and σ_{i2} are their corresponding standard deviations. A high P-metric value for a PC implies that it provides a good separation between the samples of the two classes. Therefore, the PCs were sorted based on their P-metric values in descending order and a subset of the first selected PCs were used in the classification stage.

2.4 Classification

Figure 1(b) illustrates two classification schemes that were trained with the parameters of the local PCA models. The first scheme uses the strategy proposed in [17] while the second one works based on the idea of concatenating the local PCA models' parameters. Both methodologies were implemented by making use of a subset of PCs that had been chosen in the feature selection stage. Note that, since the local PCA models were trained independently, the selected PCs for each model can be different from the others. SVM [3] with a linear kernel was used as classifier in both global and local models. Classification outcomes were achieved using 10-fold cross-validation. Hereto, data vectors were randomly divided into 10 equal-size folds such that each fold had the same number of patterns from each class. Classifiers were trained with the first nine folds and tested with the last one. This procedure was repeated 10 times so that all folds were used for training and testing the classifiers.

3 Results

Average classification outcomes obtained with the global PCA model are shown in Fig. 2. While the best result of the classifier trained with the first PCs

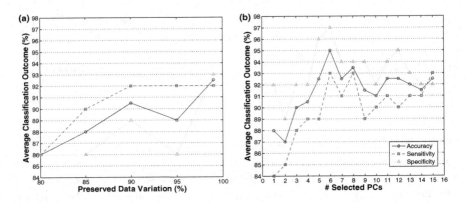

Fig. 2. Average classification outcomes (%) with the global PCA model. (a) Training the classifier with a subset of the first PCs or (b) with a subset of the selected PCs.

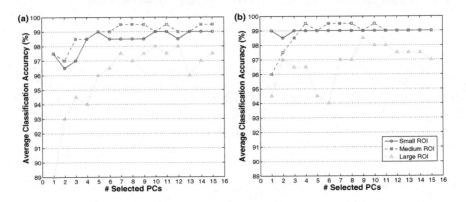

Fig. 3. Average classification accuracies (%) obtained with the selected PCs of the local PCA models and utilizing (a) the classifier voting scheme and (b) the proposed classification framework.

Table 1. Best average classification accuracies (%) and their corresponding sensitivity and specificity values obtained with the global PCA model (typed in bold). The (min,max) ranges of the obtained outcomes are also presented.

	Accuracy	Sensitivity	Specificity
First PCs	**92.5** (80,100)	**92** (80,100)	**93** (80,100)
Selected PCs	95 (80,100)	93 (80,100)	97 (80,100)

(Fig. 2(a)) was achieved by preserving 99% of the data variation (the first 60 PCs), training the classifier with the selected PCs (Fig. 2(b)) yielded better performance with considerably less number of features (6 PCs).

Table 2. Best average classification accuracies (%) and their corresponding sensitivity and specificity values obtained with the local PCA models (typed in bold). The (min,max) ranges of the obtained outcomes are also presented.

	Accuracy	Sensitivity	Specificity
Classifier Voting Scheme			
Small ROI	**99** (95,100)	**98** (90,100)	**100** (100,100)
Medium ROI	**99.5** (95,100)	**99** (90,100)	**100** (100,100)
Large ROI	**98** (90,100)	**98** (90,100)	**98** (90,100)
The proposed Scheme			
Small ROI	**99** (95,100)	**98** (90,100)	**100** (100,100)
Medium ROI	**99.5** (95,100)	**99** (90,100)	**100** (100,100)
Large ROI	**98.5** (95,100)	**97** (90,100)	**100** (100,100)

Figure 3 illustrates the average classification accuracies achieved by the local PCA models. It can be seen that all local models could provide significantly higher classification results than the global ones. The best classification results of the global and local PCA models along with their corresponding sensitivity and specificity values are listed in Tables 1 and 2, respectively.

In order to give insight into the characteristics of the selected PCs that enable a classifier to discriminate between the normal and infarcted LV shapes, the first five selected modes of variation of the global PCA model, which were observed constantly across the 10 folds, are visualized in Fig. 4. Note that the reason for visualizing the global PCs is that they are easier to interpret than the local PCs.

4   Discussion

4.1   Global Versus Local Statistical Modeling

It has been demonstrated that by using a limited number of the landmark points, a local framework is able to provide better statistical description of LV shapes than its global counterpart. The performance of the local structures, however, depends on the ROI size and tuning this parameter needs a proper compromise between the statistical significance and number of landmark points. Although the performance of the local classification schemes in detecting myocardial infarction is comparable, direct usage of the local models' parameters and considering the spatial relation between the LV segments would enable the proposed scheme to properly deal with different abnormalities that affect small regions of the myocardium.

As shown in Fig. 3, the favorable results of the classifier voting and the proposed scheme were obtained by using a few number of selected PCs per local PCA model which can be explained by the following reasons: (1) local regions have less modes of variation than the whole LV and their statistical modeling

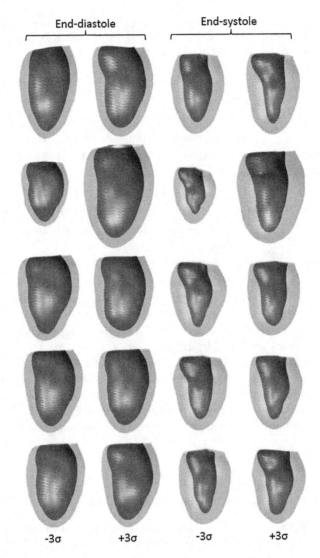

Fig. 4. Variations of the first five selected PCs of the global PCA model at end-diastole and end-systole. From top, PCs 18, 1, 20, 42 and 15 are the selected modes of variation.

needs less number of components as well, (2) as shown in Fig. 2(b), selected PCs could provide considerable discriminatory information for the local classification systems.

4.2   Feature Selection Utility

The obtained results confirm the suitability of the feature selection strategy where training a classifier with a small group of the selected PCs could significantly enhance the performance of the same classifier that was trained with a much larger subset of the first PCs. To shed further light on the utility of the feature selection method and statistical shape modeling with PCA, some patho-physiological interpretations of the selected PCs belong to the global PCA model (shown in Fig. 4) are given in the following.

The left- and righ-hand sides of each LV mode in Fig. 4 correspond to the anteroseptal and inferolateral walls, respectively. The first selected mode (PC 18) describes variations in the curvature of the anterior wall. This PC might have been selected also due to possible difference in contouring convention of the left ventricular outflow tract (LVOT) in the MESA and DETERMINE trials. The second selected mode (PC 1) explains variations in the LV size. Blunting of the apex and variation of the inferior wall curvature is described by the third selected mode (PC 20). The forth selected mode (PC 42) is associated with the end-systolic variations in the curvatures of the inferior region and the anterior wall. Finally, the fifth selected mode (PC 15) captures the rightward shifting of the apex and variations in the inferior region.

The above-mentioned patho-physiological interpretations are mostly based on the evidences presented in [4, 11] and are associated with the process of the LV remodeling due to anterior myocardial infarction. Although the DETERMINE study involves patients with different types of the myocardial infarction, it is well-known that coronary artery disease occurs most commonly in the left anterior descending (LAD) coronary artery. Therefore, interpretation of the selected PCs based on the findings of [4, 11] might be valid for the majority of the subjects in this study.

5   Conclusion

A statistical framework has been established based on local PCA models to characterize major modes of LV shape variation. Although local statistical modeling could bring favorable advantages over global parametrization, the adopted strategy for associating the local models' parameters plays a key role in obtaining an efficient local-to-global shape characterization. We hypothesized that the concatenation of the local models' parameters would lead to such efficient characterization. Parameters of each local model were selected based on their significance in discriminating normal and infarcted shapes. Classification outcomes confirmed the superiority of the proposed statistical framework over the global model. They also approved the suitability of the feature selection strategy where utilizing a few number of selected PCs could yield high classification results.

References

1. Bild, D.E., Bluemke, D.A., Burke, G.L., Detrano, R., Roux, A.V.D., et al.: Multiethnic study of atherosclerosis: objectives and design. Am. J. Epidemiol. **156**, 871–881 (2002)

2. Cootes, T.F., Cooper, D., Taylor, C.J., Graham, J.: Active shape models-their training and application. Comput. Vis. Image Understand. **61**(1), 38–59 (1995)
3. Cristianini, N., Shawe-Taylore, J.: An Introduction to Support Vector Machines. Cambridge University Press, Cambridge (2000)
4. Di Donato, M., Dabic, P., Castelvecchio, S., Santambrogio, C., Brankovic, J., Collarini, L., et al.: Left ventricular geometry in normal and post-anterior myocardial infarction patients: sphericity index and new conicity index comparisons. Eur. J. Cardio-Thorac. Surg. **29**, S225–S230 (2006)
5. Roohi, S., Zoroofi, R.: 4D statistical shape modeling of the left ventricle in cardiac MR images. Int. J. CARS **8**, 335–351 (2013)
6. Fonseca, C.G., Backhaus, M., Bluemke, D.A., Britten, R.D., Do Chung, J., Cowan, B.R., Dinov, I.D., Fin, J.P., Hunter, P.J., Kadish, A.H., Lee, D.C., Lima, J.A., Medrano-Gracia, P., Shivkumar, K., Suinesiaputra, A., Tao, W., Young, A.A.: The Cardiac Atlas Project - an imaging database for computational modeling and statistical atlases of the heart. Bioinformatics **27**(16), 2288–2295 (2011)
7. Frangi, A.F., Rueckert, D., Schnabel, J.A., Niessen, W.J.: Automatic construction of multiple-object three-dimensional statistical shape models: application to cardiac modeling. IEEE Trans. Med. Imaging **21**(9), 1151–1164 (2002)
8. Inza, I., Larranaga, P., Blanco, R., Cerrolaza, A.J.: Filter versus wrapper gene selection approaches in DNA microarray domains. Artif. Intell. Med. **31**, 91–103 (2004)
9. Jolliffe, I.T.: Principal Component Analysis. Springer, New York (1986)
10. Kadish, A.H., Bello, D., Finn, J., Bonow, R.O., Schaechter, A., Subacius, H., Albert, C., Daubert, J.P., Fonseca, C.G., Goldberger, J.J.: Rationale and design for the defibrillators to reduce risk by magnetic resonance imaging evaluation (DETERMINE) trial. J. Cardiovas. Electrophysiol. **20**, 982–987 (2009)
11. Mitchell, G.F., Lamas, G.A., Vaughan, D.E., Pfeffer, M.A.: Left ventricular remodeling in the year after first anterior myocardial infarction: a quantitative analysis of contractile segment lengths and ventricular shape. J. Am. Coll. Cardiol. **19**(6), 1136–1144 (1992)
12. Perperidis, D., Mohiaddin, R.H., Rueckert, D.: Construction of a 4D statistical atlas of the cardiac anatomy and its use in classification. In: Duncan, J.S., Gerig, G. (eds.) MICCAI 2005. LNCS, vol. 3750, pp. 402–410. Springer, Heidelberg (2005)
13. Rohlf, F., Slice, D.: Extensions of the procrustus method for the optimal superimposition of landmarks. Syst. Zool. **39**, 40–59 (1990)
14. Stegmann, M.B., Stojstrand, K., Larsen, R.: Sparse modeling of landmark and texture variability using the orthomax criterion. In: International Symposium on Medical Imaging, vol. 6144, pp. 485–496 (2006)
15. Suinesiaputra, A., Frangi, A.F., Kaandorp, T.A.M., Lamb, H.J., Bax, J.J., Reiber, J.H.C., Lelieveldt, B.P.F.: Automated detection of regional wall motion abnormalities based on a statistical model applied to multislice short-axis cardiac MR images. IEEE Trans. Med. Imaging **28**(4), 595–607 (2009)
16. Tenenbaum, J.B., De Silva, V., Langford, J.C.: A global geometric framework for nonlinear dimensionality reduction. Science **290**, 2319–2323 (2000)
17. Ye, D.H., Desjardins, B., Hamm, J., Litt, H., Pohl, K.M.: Regional manifold learning for disease classification. IEEE Trans. Med. Imaging **33**(6), 1236–1247 (2014)
18. Zhang, X., Cowan, B.R., Bluemke, D.A., Finn, J.P., Fonseca, C.G., Kadish, A.H., Lee, D.C., Lima, J.A.C., Suinesiaputra, A., Young, A.A., Medrano-Gracia, P.: Atlas-based quantification of cardiac remodeling due to myocardial infarction. PLOS ONE **9**(10), e110243 (2014)

Erratum to: Myocardial Infarction Detection from Left Ventricular Shapes Using a Random Forest

Jack Allen[1(✉)], Ernesto Zacur[2], Erica Dall'Armellina[1], Pablo Lamata[2], and Vicente Grau[1]

[1] University of Oxford, Oxford, UK
jack.allen@jesus.ox.ac.uk
[2] King's College London, London, UK

Erratum to:
Chapter 20: O. Camara et al. (Eds.)
Statistical Atlases and Computational Models of the Heart,
DOI: 10.1007/978-3-319-28712-6_20

The following acknowledgement was omitted from the paper entitled "Myocardial Infarction Detection from Left Ventricular Shapes Using a Random Forest"

Acknowledgements. This work was supported by funding from the Medical Research Council (MRC) and Engineering and Physical Sciences Research Council (EPSRC) [grant number EP/L016052/1].

The updated original online version for this chapter can be found at
10.1007/978-3-319-28712-6_20

Author Index